# MASSAGE THERAPY MEDICAL REPORTS

# MASSAGE THERAPY MEDICAL REPORTS

NAEEM SHARIEFF

Copyright © 2012 by Naeem Sharieff.

| Library of Congress Control Number: | | 2012902264 |
|---|---|---|
| ISBN: | Hardcover | 978-1-4691-6366-6 |
| | Softcover | 978-1-4691-6365-9 |
| | Ebook | 978-1-4691-6367-3 |

All rights reserved. No part of this book may be reproduced or transmitted in any form or by any means, electronic or mechanical, including photocopying, recording, or by any information storage and retrieval system, without permission in writing from the copyright owner.

This book was printed in the United States of America.

To order additional copies of this book, contact:
Xlibris Corporation
1-888-795-4274
www.Xlibris.com
Orders@Xlibris.com
110355

# Contents

Acupressure Specialist Evaluation ................................................................. 1
Alternative Medicine AOE / COE Evaluation ................................................ 5
Back Pain Report ............................................................................................. 11
Brief Progress Report ...................................................................................... 14
Carpal Tunnel Report ..................................................................................... 16
Cervical Spine Report ..................................................................................... 18
Clinical Consultation Evaluation ................................................................... 20
Clinical Consultation Report ......................................................................... 29
Equine Massage Therapy Report ................................................................... 36
Explosion Medical Report .............................................................................. 39
Facial Paralysis Report .................................................................................... 42
Follow-Up Report ............................................................................................ 46
Headache Report ............................................................................................. 48
Independent Medical Exam ........................................................................... 51
Initial Acupressure Report ............................................................................. 54
Jaw Pain Report ............................................................................................... 60
Left Knee Report .............................................................................................. 64
Left-Side Paralysis Report .............................................................................. 67
Left Wrist Report ............................................................................................. 71
Lower-Back Pain Report ................................................................................. 75
Lumbar Spine Report ...................................................................................... 78
Multiple Injuries Report ................................................................................. 80
Neck Pain Report ............................................................................................ 83
Neck and Shoulder Pain Report .................................................................... 86
Patient Progress Report .................................................................................. 89
Review of Records ........................................................................................... 94
Right-Side Paralysis Report ............................................................................ 98
Thoracic Spine Report .................................................................................... 100
Whole Body Paralysis ...................................................................................... 101
Bonus Templates .............................................................................................. 105

# Alien Pain Care Clinic ™

336 Huge Tree Street, West Hills, CA 91307     Tel: (818) 000-1234

---

October 02, 2011

Attention: Dr. Hamid Mir, MD

       Regarding:       Eric Baraka
       SSN:       xxx-xx-1234
       Employer:       National Cement Factory
       Insurance:       Freeway Insurance
       Claim No:       FI 06879323-WC-01
       WCAB No:       VNO 0587088, ADJ 7896542
       Date of Injury:       CT 04/08/2009 to 08/24/2010

## ACUPRESSURE SPECIALIST EVALUATION

This report has been produced for the use in the labor court proceedings of this patient and should not be used in any other proceedings such as civil and federal courts.

Dear Gentlepersons:

Eric Baraka was initially seen in my office on September 15, 2011. I have personally taken the patient's interview and performed the physical examination. Rosemary, a certified interpreter, was present.

## JOB DESCRIPTION

The patient is a fifty-one-year-old Hispanic male who worked for National Cement Factory for four years as a truck driver. He worked eight to twelve hours a day, six days a week. He is still on the above-mentioned company's payroll. His last day of work was 08/24/10. He is currently on disability by his primary treating physician, Dr. Hamid Mir. The patient has not worked since then.

## HISTORY OF INJURY

The patient was cleaning the truck, which was one of his duties. He had to lift the chute to clean the truck. Two times while working for the above company, he did this, and he injured his lower back and right shoulder. First one occurred in 2009, and second one in 2010. The patient reported these injuries to his supervisor, Edward Dinaro, who sent him to a company's doctor. Dr. Hamid Mir treated this patient and referred to this office for pain treatment.

The patient is in constant pain since April 2009. He takes pain medication and physical therapy and is waiting for right shoulder surgery. The patient has no preexisting knowledge of hypertension. He had seen a doctor on April 2009 after the first injury where he was diagnosed with hypertension and was started on medication. At the same time, he is taking pain pills and starting to develop palpitations. The patient states that he still gets palpitations on a daily basis. It comes on its own.

At times, he is woken up from sleep by the palpitations and pain. When he gets the palpitation, he gets shortness of breath and chest pain. The patient has not gained weight. The patient has the following problems with ADL (active daily living): moderate problems with bathing, dressing oneself, riding, standing, sitting, reclining, walking, climbing stairs, kneeling, driving, and sleeping. The patient has problems in sleeping due to pain and palpitations.

## PRESENT SYMPTOMS

1. Low-back pain—constant to moderate
2. Right shoulder pain—constant to moderate
3. Palpitations—constant to moderate
4. Shortness of breath—constant to moderate
5. Chest pain—constant to moderate
6. Insomnia

## CURRENT MEDICAL HISTORY

The patient is currently treated by Dr. Hamid Mir and Dr. Tabraz, who put him on disability.

## PAST MEDICAL HISTORY

The patient injured his right shoulder ten years ago and filed a workers' compensation case and recovered. He had a clavicle surgery, finger amputation surgery, and appendectomy. The patient states that he was in another job in Europe when the finger was cut off during his operation of a butcher machine in a meat shop. The patient states that he has a past history of hypertension.

## ALLERGIES

The patient denies allergies to food, medication, or environmental agents.

## MEDICATION

The patient takes sleep medication.

## SOCIAL HISTORY

The patient denies smoking, drinking, or illicit drug use.

## FAMILY HISTORY

Noncontributory

## PAST OCCUPATIONAL HISTORY

Noncontributory

## PHYSICAL EXAMINATION

| | |
|---|---|
| Height: | 5 ft. 9 in. |
| Weight: | 220 lb. |

| | |
|---|---|
| Blood pressure: | 150/100 |
| Pulse: | 88 |
| Temperature: | 97.8 |
| Skin: | Tattoos |
| Upper Extremities: | Right middle finger amputation |

## RECOMMENDATION

Twenty-four-hour blood pressure monitoring to find out the patient's hypertension, complaints of palpitations, and stress; echocardiogram to see any signs of vascular disease or disorder.

The patient should be reevaluated by a cardiologist after abovementioned testing.

Furthermore, I would recommend him for twenty sessions of martial arts medical massage, twice a week for ten weeks to get good results. This would indeed help him out for relief from pain and discomfort and improves his general health.

## PLEASE NOTE

Labor Code 5402 (c) requires the employer to authorize all appropriate medical care up to $10,000 until the liability for the claimed injury is accepted or rejected. As of 06/01/2004, Labor Code section 5814 mandates a 25 percent penalty on the amount of payment unreasonably delayed (10 percent if self-imposed). Accordingly, it would be requested that the defendant please provide immediate payment.

## DISCLOSURE

I declare under penalty of perjury that the information contained in this report and its attachments, if any, are true and correct to the best of my knowledge and belief.

———————————————

DR. NAEEM SHARIEFF
*Acupressure Specialist*

# Alien Pain Care Clinic ™

336 Huge Tree Street, West Hills, CA 91307　　　　Tel: (818) 000-1234

---

October 05, 2011

City of Hope
Workers Compensation Division
789 W. Bumpy Street, Room 110
City of Hope, CA 90077

Attention: Ms. Dona Pratt, Claim Adjuster

| | |
|---|---|
| Regarding: | Sam Ramos |
| SSN: | xxx-xx-1234 |
| Employer: | City of Hope |
| Insurance: | Runners Insurance |
| Claim No: | RI 06878328-WC-011 |
| WCAB No: | VNO 0577088, ADJ 7746542 |
| Date of Injury: | 06/30/10 |

## ALTERNATIVE MEDICINE AOE / COE EVALUATION

This report has been produced for the use in the labor court proceedings of this patient and should not be used in any other proceedings, such as civil and federal courts.

## INTRODUCTION

Mr. Sam Ramos, a forty-five-year-old Hispanic male, was seen at my office as indicated above and examined personally by me today. This acupressure therapy evaluation was performed at his request for the purpose of obtaining my opinion as an acupressure specialist regarding an injury claim arising out of Mr. Ramos's employment with the City of Hope. The following is a summary of this patient's current status and findings.

**CHIEF COMPLAINT**

This forty-five-year-old telecom associate is seen for evaluation of discomfort in his low back.

**HISTORY OF PRESENT INJURY**

The patient states that he had the gradual onset of discomfort in his lower back and did not have a specific injury. His symptoms began in early June 2005. He developed back discomfort after sitting at work. His discomfort improved when he went home and after a night's rest. His symptoms would return the following day after prolonged sitting. He sought medical care with his HMO, and he was given medication including analgesics and anti-inflammatory medication. The patient was seen in consultation by Dr. William and was treated with oral steroids, which did not improve his symptoms.

The patient sought medical treatment with a chiropractor on July 18, 2010, and received chiropractic treatment five days a week. He states that these treatments helped temporarily. His symptoms are relieved by taking medication.

In general, the patient feels that his symptoms are worsening. The patient states that prior to June 2008, he had daily symptoms of discomfort in the right lower extremity. He noted that since the onset of his back pain. His symptoms have been present especially after driving long distances.

**CURRENT COMPLAINTS**

Currently, the patient states that he has constant low-back discomfort and a feeling of stiffness. He states that he has no difficulty with back movements and he has no radiating pain from the low back. He states he has numbness and tingling extending down his leg to the lateral aspect of his foot. He is occasionally awakened with night pain. He does not have true pain in the right leg, but only has numbness and tingling. The patient's back discomfort is located low in the back and in the buttocks bilaterally.

## PAST MEDICAL HISTORY

The patient states that he had back discomfort in March 2007, which lasted three months. He was seen by a private physician. The patient's symptoms were resolved. There was no time lost from work.

## EMPLOYMENT HISTORY

This patient is currently working at his usual and customary occupation as a telecom associate. His duties require two to three hours of data entry, sitting, and writing. He also drives to different locations to do network design and site survey. He does no lifting. The patient has been employed for seven years by his present employer and has a very good attendance record.

## PHYSICAL EXAMINATION

The patient is 5 ft. 6 in. tall and weighs 180 lb. He does not appear to be in acute distress. He appears to be in a satisfactory state of health.

Examination of the lumbar spine reveals no evidence of paravertebral muscle spasm. The patient has slight laxity of the abdominal muscles. He has a normal lumbar curve. There was no tenderness to palpation in the midline of the lumbar spine. He had slight tenderness bilaterally over the posterior superior iliac spine. Full range of motion was accomplished without discomfort. There was no dysrhythmia. No paravertebral muscle spasm occurred after range of motion.

Sitting straight-leg raising was negative. Recumbent straight-leg raising was carried to ninety degrees bilaterally. Lasegue's sign revealed no hamstrings tightness. Hip flexion did not produce low-back discomfort.

Neurologic examination revealed equal, deep tendon reflexes and there was no motor weakness. The patient had decreased sensation over the S1 dermatome of the right foot.

Examination of the abdomen reveals that the patient is able to perform a weak half sit-up without discomfort. The patient was comfortable in the prone position and could perform a back extension without discomfort.

## ROENTGENOGRAMS

Films of the lumbar spine were examined by Dr. Mohsen, who is a certified radiologist. According to him, lumbar spine reveals slight anterior wedging at T12 and L1, suggestive of old juvenile epiphysitis. Disk heights are well preserved at all levels. The patient had an intact lumbar lordotic curve. Oblique views revealed no pars defects. Sacroiliac joints were normal.

## DIAGNOSIS

Low-back pain of unknown etiology.

## DISCUSSION

This patient states that he has constant low-back discomfort, which began in June 2005. The patient was having preexisting symptoms in the right lower extremity of numbness and tingling, and this has continued since the onset of his low-back discomfort. These symptoms follow the S1 nerve distribution. His physical examination reveals no abnormality in regard to the lumbar spine aside from sensory change involving the S1 dermatome on the right.

## CAUSATION

Based on the information I have at this time, I feel that the patient's condition is nonindustrial and would be related to a preexisting condition.

## WORK RESTRICTIONS

The patient should do no sitting longer than thirty minutes without a break.

## MEDICAL TREATMENT

A lumbar MRI should be obtained.

The patient should be reevaluated by an examination after his lumbar spine MRI has been obtained.

The patient should be scheduled for martial arts medical massage in our clinic twice a week for ten weeks to relieve constant pain.

The patient should be on an abdominal exercise program to strengthen his paraspinal musculature. Some classes of yoga or a home-based exercise program is highly recommended for fitness.

## DISCLOSURE

The history contained herein was outlined by my historian, Ginger, and medical record reviewed by myself in the presence of the patient.

## END OF THE REPORT

---

DR. NAEEM SHARIEFF
*Acupressure Specialist*

PROOF OF SERVICE ATTACHED

# PROOF OF SERVICE BY MAIL

STATE OF CALIFORNIA, COUNTY OF LOS ANGELES

I am a resident of the county aforesaid, and I am over the age of eighteen years and not a party to the within action. My business address is 336 Huge Tree Street, West Hills, CA 91307.

On October 05, 2011, I served the within concerning:

> Patient Name:  Sam Ramos
> Claim No:  RI 06878328-WC-011
> WCAB No:  VNO 0577088, ADJ 7746542

On the interested parties in said action, by placing a true copy thereof enclosed in a sealed envelope with postage thereon fully prepaid in Los Angeles, California.

- ☐ Medical Lien
- ☐ Medical Report
- ☐ Doctor's First Report
- ☐ Patient's Progress Report
- ☐ Radiological Report
- ☐ Review of Records
- ☐ Demand Letter
- ☐ Declaration of Readiness to Proceed
- ☐ Trial Brief / Exhibits
- ☐ Hearing Notice
- ☐ Workers Compensation Lien
- ☐ Initial Report
- ☐ Reevaluation Report
- ☐ Permanent and Stationary Report
- ☐ AME / QME Report
- ☐ Itemized Billing Statement / HFCA
- ☐ Lien Settlement Agreement
- ☐ Withdrawal of DOR
- ☐ Stipulation and Order
- ☐ Excuse to Attend Hearing

**Parties served:**

Law Offices of Choti Ghulail
3378 Victory Blvd.
West Hills, CA 91307

I declare under penalty and perjury under the laws of the State of California, that the foregoing is true and correct, and that this declaration was executed at Los Angeles, California on October 5, 2011.

---

KENNETH VILLA

# East Coast Back Pain Clinic

333 Grand Trunk Road  
Williamsville, Buffalo, NY 91441

Tel: (201) 000-1234  
Fax: (201) 000-1235

---

Patient Name:        Willy Barillas  
SSN:                 xxx-xx-1234  
Examination:         Back Pain  
Referring Physician: Dr. Mehnaz Khan  
Examination Date:    10/05/2011  
Today's Date:        10/22/2011

## DESCRIPTION

The patient is a sixty-two-year-old male working as a full-time project manager in a local hospital and is required to do extensive walking at various periods during a workday.

## HISTORY OF INJURY

The patient was referred to physical therapy, secondary to low-back pain and degenerative disk disease. The patient states that he has had a cauterization of some sort to the nerves in his low back to help alleviate with painful symptoms. The patient would benefit from skilled physical therapy intervention.

The patient has a history of low-back pain, secondary to a fall that originally occurred in 2008. The patient states that he slipped on a newly waxed floor and fell on his tailbone and low-back region. The patient then had his second fall in April 2009. The patient states that he was qualifying on the range with a handgun and lost his footing and states that he fell more due to weakness in his lower extremities rather than loss of balance.

## PAST SURGICAL HISTORY

The patient has a past surgical history of appendectomy.

## DIAGNOSIS

Low-back pain and degenerative lumbar disk

## MEDICATIONS

The patient is taking ibuprofen 800 mg occasionally as needed for pain management.

## SOCIAL HISTORY

The patient states that he lives in a condo with his wife and a son, who are in good health and are able to assist with any task or activity the patient is having difficulty with. The patient rates his general health as excellent and denies any smoking, alcohol, and drug use.

## MEDICAL IMAGING

The patient states that he has had an MRI recently performed; however, the results are not available at the time of the evaluation. The patient states that he is able to bring the report in upon next visit.

## SUBJECTIVE COMPLAINT

The patient rates his pain at 7/10 on a pain analog scale, 0 to 10, 10 being worse. The patient describes his pain as a deep aching, primarily on the right lower back and gluteal region. Aggravating factors include stairs and prolonged driving, as well as general limitations with home tasks and projects. The patient states he is a very active individual and is noticing extreme limitations with ability to complete home tasks and projects he used to be able to complete.

## NEUROLOGICAL SYMPTOMS

The patient reports having occasional shooting pains into the lower extremities. However, these are occurring less frequently and are now occurring more frequently in the right versus the left lower extremity when they do occur.

## ACTIVE RANGE OF MOTION OF LUMBAR SPINE

Forward flexion is 26 cm, fingertip to floor; lateral side bend, fingertip to floor, is 52.5 cm bilaterally.

## STRENGTH

Strength is grossly 4/5. The patient denies any significant tenderness to palpation. However, does have mild increase in tenderness on the right versus left. A six-minute walk test revealed painful symptoms and achiness occurring after approximately four hundred feet of walking. The patient was able to continue; however, stopped after seven hundred feet. There were two minutes remaining in the six-minute walk test. The patient does have tight hamstrings as well as a negative slump test.

## TREATMENT PLAN

The patient to be seen three times a week for six weeks for the following:

1. Therapeutic exercise with home exercise program.
2. Modalities to include ice, heat, ultrasound, electrical stimulation in order to reduce pain and inflammation.
3. Manual therapy to include soft tissue mobilization and joint mobilization as needed in order to promote increased mobility and decreased muscle tightness.

I have discussed the plan of care with the patient as well as the findings of the evaluation. The patient reports understanding and agrees to be compliant with physical therapy intervention.

---

MARIA ARRIYOLA, LMT

# Brief Progress Report

From:_____

To:_____

Progress Report as of:___/___/___

Regarding:_____

Treatments since last report:_____

Current Rx expires:_____

Overall Patient Progress: ___Poor ___Marginal ___Good ___Excellent

Areas Treated: __Cervical __Thoracic __Lumbar __Sacral __Other

## SUBJECTIVE AND OBJECTIVE OBSERVATIONS

|  | Left | Right | No Current Problem | Improving | Not Improving | Increased Symptoms |
|---|---|---|---|---|---|---|
| **Neck** |  |  |  |  |  |  |
| **Shoulder** |  |  |  |  |  |  |
| **Arm** |  |  |  |  |  |  |
| **Midback** |  |  |  |  |  |  |
| **Low Back** |  |  |  |  |  |  |
| **Pelvis** |  |  |  |  |  |  |
| **Knee** |  |  |  |  |  |  |
| **Leg** |  |  |  |  |  |  |

Brief Progress Report

Patient stress level rate: \_\_\_ Low  \_\_\_ Moderate  \_\_\_ High

Other: _____

Comment: _____
_____
_____
_____

Thank you for your referral.

_____
ABEL ARROBANG, LMT

Date: _____

# NY Pain Treatment Center

108 Welcome Street　　　　　　　　　　　　　Tel: (551) 123-4567
Jersey City, NJ 07802　　　　　　　　　　　　Fax: (551) 123-4568

---

| | |
|---|---|
| Patient Name: | Brian Lee |
| SSN: | xxx-xx-1234 |
| Examination: | Carpal Tunnel Syndrome |
| Referring Physician: | Dr. Saleem Sharieff |
| Examination Date: | 07/29/2011 |
| Today's Date: | 07/31/2011 |

## PATIENT HISTORY

The patient is a thirty-five-year-old gentleman with numbness primarily in the upper extremities. This study was requested to evaluate for carpal tunnel syndrome.

## SUBJECTIVE COMPLAINTS

Exacerbated pain level. Handicap due to pain. Increased pain in arms and hand. Significant difficulty to sleep. Patient feels very anxious/stressed regarding job activities.

## OBJECTIVE FINDINGS

Patient reported significant pain in wrist / carpal tunnel syndrome with numbness and tingling.

## IMPRESSION

There are no additional findings to support a diagnosis of carpal tunnel syndrome as tested on the right side.

## IMPROVEMENT

Progressing with treatment. Decrease in handicap. Patient notes general decrease in severity of pain, weakness, numbness, and tingling.

Thank you for referring this patient.

_____

AULINE ARROBANG, LMT

# Alien Pain Care Clinic ™

105 Welcome Street, New Jersey, NJ 07802      Tel: (551) 000-0000

---

|  |  |
|---|---|
| Patient Name: | Marina Nehorayan |
| SSN: | xxx-xx-1234 |
| Examination: | Cervical Spine |
| Referring Physician: | Dr. Iqbal Karimullah |
| Examination Date: | 06/13/2011 |
| Today's Date: | 07/24/2011 |

Manual therapy for pain control.

## CLINICAL HISTORY

Neck pain.

## TECHNIQUE

Martial arts medical massage was performed in chronic pain with the use of elbow, fingers, fist, and knuckles. The following methods were not used in this therapy:

no electrical devices, no mechanical devices, no needles, no medications, no heat pad, no cold pad, no heat lamp, no rollers and balls, no oil or lotion, no stone, no cupping, no magnets, no traction, no laser, and no ultrasound.

## FINDINGS

No obvious abnormality noted.

## IMPRESSION

Mild disk bulging.

## RECOMMENDATION

Additional testing may be helpful, if clinically desirable and appropriate, such as magnetic resonance imaging (MRI) and a home-based exercise program consisting of stretching, strengthening, and range of motion exercises. A class of yoga or tai chi is highly recommended for faster rehabilitation.

Thank you for referring this patient.

_____
EDDIE ARROBANG, CMT

## NAEEM SHARIEFF, BA, LLB, MA, MDAM
*Acupressure Specialist*
1947 Roswell Street, Suite 100
Los Angeles, CA 91335
Tel: (818) 000-0000

August 30, 2011

Timothy Mason, Esq.
99084 Roscoe Blvd., Suite 92
Agora Hills, CA 91346

Attention: Attorney Mason

| | |
|---|---|
| Regarding: | Harry Foster |
| Occupation: | Firefighter |
| Employer: | City of Los Angeles |
| Date of Injury: | CT May 17, 1999 to December 18, 2010 |
| Date of Exam: | August 30, 2011 |
| Claim Number: | 1896482 |
| WCAB Case No: | ADJ3748673, VNO 9533124 |

## CLINICAL CONSULTATION EVALUATION

## SECTIONS OF THE REPORT

| I | Parameters of the Report | Page 22 |
|---|---|---|
| II | Reason for Referral | Page 22 |
| III | Identifying Data | Page 22 |
| IV | Presenting Situation | Page 22 |
| V | Psychiatric History | Page 24 |
| VI | Past and Family History | Page 24 |
| VII | Medical History | Page 25 |
| VIII | Developmental and Educational History | Page 25 |
| IX | Personal Habits | Page 25 |
| X | Activities/Hobbies | Page 25 |
| XI | Legal Consideration | Page 25 |
| XII | Mental Status Observation | Page 26 |
| | Appearance | Page 26 |
| | Behavior | Page 26 |
| | Affect and Mood | Page 26 |
| | Thought Content | Page 26 |
| XIII | Diagnostic Impression | Page 26 |
| XIV | Clinical Syndromes | Page 27 |
| XV | Medical Opinion | Page 27 |
| XVI | Recommendations | Page 27 |
| XII | Therapeutic Consideration | Page 27 |
| XVII | Reevaluation | Page 27 |
| XIX | Declaration | Page 28 |

## PARAMETERS OF THE REPORT

Harry Foster was seen in our office for acupressure therapy and was told that he was being evaluated exclusively of his workers' compensation claim at the request of his attorney and the defendants and that no treatment relationship existed (doctor-therapist-patient) and that any information provided, as well as the results of the therapeutic testing and my conclusions regarding the case, would be included in a report that may be read by people involved in the resolution and/or litigation of his claim.

The patient stated that he understood the aforementioned and agreed to proceed with the evaluation. The report belongs to the party or parties requesting the evaluation. If the patient wishes to review this report, I prefer that he review it under the supervision of a therapist or an experienced staff member because the report may be easily misinterpreted by the patient.

## REASON FOR REFERRAL

The patient has been referred to our office for evaluation because he filed a claim alleging an emotional/work-related injury. This report will render a therapeutic opinion and the need for any therapeutic treatment.

## IDENTIFYING DATA

The patient is a fifty-four-year-old Caucasian male, 6 ft. tall, weighs 235 lb. He is fairly stocky in his appearance and has blond hair. He is casually and appropriately dressed. He is still fairly notably husky in regard to his size. The patient's employer at the time of injury is identified to be the City of Los Angeles.

## PRESENTING SITUATION
(as related by the patient)

The patient's job is a firefighter. The patient's job description and duties were associated with emergency response training station as well as equipment duties. The patient's supervisor's name was Mark Brown, captain.

The patient identifies his last day of work to be December 17, 2010. The patient is currently on leave for issues associated with heart, stress, as well as vertigo. The patient's job duties that he performed on a regular basis included sitting, standing, bending, kneeling, twisting, reaching, walking, stooping, pushing, pulling, light lifting, as well as heavy lifting. The patient indicates that his working hours were ten scheduled twenty-four-hour shifts per month plus overtime. The patient is noted to have no problems with negative write-ups, never being sent for counseling, and has no disciplinary actions. The patient identifies no suspensions. He indicates that he had always had what he indicated to be exceeding and outperforming from a standpoint of his work performance evaluations.

The patient identifies his current specific injury on July 4, 2004. The patient states that it was at that time he was at station 21, where he was involved in a training exercise, which was an emergency bailout from an upper floor. The patient states that one is supposed to head out through the window then hook themselves with their arms and essentially pivot themselves onto the ladder. The patient noted that during the exercise, they are actually in safety harnesses. The patient states that when he went out of the window, the harness got stuck on the ladder, essentially catching the patient and pulling his full weight onto his right upper extremity, swinging him out and hitting his left knee, and essentially pulling all his weight on his right upper extremity.

The patient states that it was soon thereafter he felt pain in his right upper extremity but notably had significant swelling of his knee. The patient states that about four to five hours, he was having difficulty in terms of ambulating and identifies that the knee had swollen to a point that he ultimately was referred to Valley Medical Center. There, x-rays were done. The patient states that his focus at that point seemed to be on his knee, although the patient noted that there seemed to be something wrong with his right upper extremity. The patient states that it wasn't diagnosed until approximately two weeks that the patient actually had a greenstick fracture of his right elbow. He could not recall how much time he had off from work, but he does identify that he eventually returned back to full duties.

The patient identifies that the second specific injury occurred on November 12, 2009. The patient states that at that time, he was at station 27. He was doing maintenance, which he indicates, in the vacant lot. There he was shoveling, moving some blocks around, as well as sandbagging, and he began to notice the onset of pain and swelling in his right elbow. He brought this to the attention of Captain Mark. The patient notes that although he reported injury to Captain, nothing really in particular was done; instead, the patient sought help from his primary care physician, Dr. Lateefa. Dr. Lateefa took him off work for a month. The patient states that he returned to his usual and customary duties thereafter.

The patient noted for the last several years that he was having ongoing difficulties falling asleep and insomnia due to stressful environment and that causes heart problems. He was referred by Dr. Lateefa to Dr. Zapata, who had been requesting consultation for psychiatric issues. The patient indicates that he is not currently taking medications.

## PSYCHIATRIC HISTORY

The patient indicates he had depression in 2001 and given Remeron. At the same time, he verbalized in the deposition of Dr. Max, a psychologist associated with just psychotherapy treatment. This in turn appears to have corresponding issues associated with derogatory names that the patient actually had been called for five years already, including the nickname Milkman.

The patient has no family members that suffer any psychiatric or psychological problems. He has never been a victim of physical or sexual abuse.

## PAST AND FAMILY HISTORY

He was originally born in Riverside, California. His upbringing was pretty typical. His mom and dad married throughout the course of their lives. Mom and dad are still living in Riverside. His mom is eighty-five. Her health is fair to poor. As noted, she does have a history of atrial fibrillation. The patient indicates that she was a homemaker. His father is now retired. He was a mechanic. The patient notes that he is eighty-eight and is fairly in good health. The patient identifies that he has fifty-one- and fifty-six-year-old brothers and a forty-five-year-old sister. The factor with his family is not a factor that has any kind of issue that has created any depression or stress for him. The patient identifies that he has a good relationship with his brothers and sister.

The patient was married from 1985 to 1998. He has no children from this marriage and no girlfriend thereafter. His breakup was due to irreconcilable differences.

## MEDICAL HISTORY

The patient had been in good health prior to the time associated with the types of injuries that the patient has endured associated with his work as a firefighter. He has undergone prior surgical procedures due to dirt bike accident as he fell off his dirt bike. He had significant injury to his left knee. The patient had at least two occasions where he was exposed to mold or toxic substance.

## DEVELOPMENTAL AND EDUCATIONAL HISTORY

The patient attended Riverside High School and graduated in 1986. He had no problems in regard to requiring any special classes or assistance. He had no problems paying attention in school. The patient identifies that he thereafter went directly into studying fire science at Santa Anita College from 1986 to 1989.

## PERSONAL HABITS

The patient himself has never had any problems with drugs or alcohol now or in the past.

## ACTIVITIES/HOBBIES

The patient identifies his excitement, and he has always enjoyed motorcycles, camping, as well as hiking and skiing. He sits around the house occasionally and watches TV or surfs the Internet.

## LEGAL CONSIDERATIONS

He has never been involved in any lawsuit except a small claims judgment in 1983, which was vacated. The patient identifies no history of jail or prison. No history of drunk driving. No financial difficulties. No history of bankruptcies. The patient indicates that his current means of support is sick leave. He gets a paycheck, which is injury on disability. This has been the current means of support at this time.

## MENTAL STATUS OBSERVATION

### APPEARANCE

(mentioned above in identifying data)

### BEHAVIOR

His facial expressions show anxiety and apprehension. His quality of speech and tone increased and decreased, depending upon issues discussed, and becomes tearful and labile during corresponding parts of the interview. In the doctor-therapist-patient relationship, he is cooperative and is not provocative or suspicious.

### AFFECT AND MOOD

The patient's mood is described as depressed. His affect shows him to be notably dysphonic and anxious. It is moderate.

### THOUGHT CONTENT

The patient's attention shows slight distractibility. His thought content shows no obsession or depersonalization. No suicidal or homicidal ideation.

### DIAGNOSTIC IMPRESSION

1. Anxiety disorder
2. Depressive disorder
3. Sleep disorder
4. Psychological factors affecting general medical condition
5. Increase in muscle tension
6. Cardiovascular issues
7. Occupational injury

## CLINICAL SYNDROMES

A major depression characterizes the daily life of this melancholic and moody man. He is filled with self-pity, feels empty and apprehensive—plagued by doubts, expecting the worst, and repeatedly undoing opportunities to better his circumstances. His mood has little reason to lift.

## MEDICAL OPINION

Although the patient himself perceives that he may be suffering from post-traumatic stress, I do not believe that he has formal post-traumatic stress, but this is indeed a stress-and-strain case over a duration and time being a firefighter. His depression is multifactorial. Based on given history and available medical records, it is my belief that the patient remain temporarily totally disabled until he maximizes medical improvement.

## RECOMMENDATIONS

It is my recommendation that the patient may have psychiatric and psychological examination before any alternative treatment. A referral should be made for such intervention and treatment on an industrial basis. He also needs *kung fu acupressure therapy* twice a week for ten weeks to improve his general health condition. There are no risk and issue associated with this therapy. This may help reducing his anxiety, depression, stress, strain, and sleep disorders.

## THERAPEUTIC CONSIDERATIONS

A time-limited and supportive therapy is needed to improve the symptoms of stress and depression, such as yoga, tai chi, acupressure, acupuncture, martial arts medical massage, and group therapy to gain his lost confidence and self-respect.

## REEVALUATION

This is a one-time consultation evaluation.

## DECLARATION

I declare that the information provided herein is true and correct to the best of my knowledge and belief.

_____

DR. NAEEM SHARIEFF
*Acupressure Specialist*

Executed at Los Angeles, California
Date: August 30, 2011

**NAEEM SHARIEFF, BA, LLB, MA, MDAM**
*Acupressure Specialist*
1947 Roswell Street, Suite 100
Los Angeles, CA 91307
Tel: (818) 000-0000

October 05, 2011

Anthony Baron, Esq.
8088 Parthia Street, Suite 142
Beverly Hills, CA 90046

Attention: Attorney Baron

| | |
|---|---|
| Regarding: | Karachi Apache |
| Employer: | City of Los Angeles |
| Date of Injury: | CT May 17, 1999 |
| Date of Exam: | August 30, 2011 |
| Examination: | Lumbar Spine HNP |

## CLINICAL CONSULTATION REPORT

### DESCRIPTION

Low-back pain and right lower-extremity pain—lumbar spine herniated nucleus pulposus.

### CHIEF COMPLAINT

Low-back pain and right lower-extremity pain. The encounter reason for today's consultation is for a second opinion regarding evaluation and treatment of the aforementioned symptoms.

### LUMBAR SPINE

The patient is a forty-two-year-old male. The current problem began about four months ago. The symptoms were sudden in onset. According to the patient, the current problem is a result of a fall. The date of injury was four months ago. There is no significant history of previous spine problems. Medical attention has been obtained through the referral source. Medical testing for the current problem includes no recent tests. Treatment for the current problem includes the following: activity modification, bracing, medications, and work modification. The following types of medications are currently being used for the present spine problem: narcotics, nonsteroidal anti-inflammatories, and muscle relaxants. The following types of medications have been used in the past: steroids. In general, the current spine problem is much worse since its onset.

## PAST SPINE HISTORY

Normal.

## PRESENT LUMBAR SYMPTOMS

Pain location: lower lumbar. The patient describes the pain as sharp. The pain ranges from none to severe. The pain is severe frequently. It is present intermittently and most of the time daily. The pain is made worse by flexion, lifting, twisting, riding in a car, and sitting. The pain is made better by laying in the supine position, medications, bracing, and rest. Sleep alteration because of pain: wakes up after getting to sleep frequently and difficulty getting to sleep frequently. Pain distribution: the lower-extremity pain is greater than the low-back pain. The patient's low-back pain appears to be discogenic in origin. The pain is much worse since its onset.

## PRESENT RIGHT LEG SYMPTOMS

Pain location: S1 dermatome (see the pain diagram). The patient describes the pain as sharp. The severity of the pain ranges from none to severe. The pain is severe frequently. It is present intermittently and most of the time daily. The pain is made worse by the same things that make the low-back pain worse. The pain is made better by the same things that make the low-back pain better. Sleep alteration because of pain: wakes up frequently after getting to sleep and difficulty getting to sleep frequently. The patient's symptoms appear to be radicular in origin. The pain is much worse since its onset.

## PAIN DIAGRAM

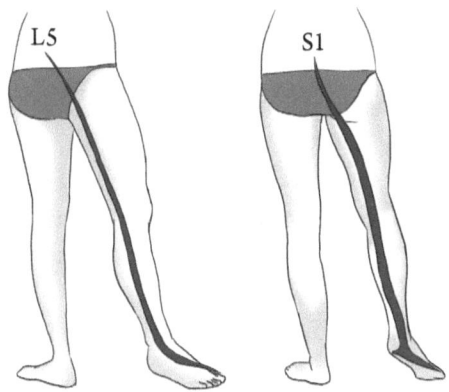

## PRESENT LEFT LEG SYMPTOMS

None.

## NEUROLOGIC SIGNS/SYMPTOMS

The patient denies any neurologic signs/symptoms. Bowel and bladder function are reported as normal. Sexual function is within normal limits.

## PAST MEDICAL HISTORY

Normal.

## PAST PSYCHE HISTORY

Unremarkable.

## PAST SURGICAL HISTORY

None.

## SOCIAL HISTORY

Occupation: Taxi driver.

Work status: On sick leave.
Marital status: Married.
Children: Two (a boy and a girl)

The patient lives at home with family.

Tobacco history: Smokes two packs of cigarettes per day. The patient denies the use of any alcoholic beverages. The patient denies any current or past history of drugs or addiction.

Family history: There are no known medical illnesses in the present and past family history.

## CURRENT GENERAL MEDICATIONS

None.

## CURRENT SPINE MEDICATIONS

Lortab 7.5, Soma, and Daypro.

## ALLERGIES

None.

## GENERAL EXAM

Mental status: normal, good historian, and normal speech.

Obesity: none.

General appearance: well developed, well nourished, normal affect, and healthy appearance.

Personality: pleasant and cooperative.

Movement about the examining room: normal with evident pain and gets in and out of a chair with difficulty.

Gait: antalgic and walks with a limp.
Heel walking: normal
Toe walking: normal
Floor squat: normal with pain
General strength: normal

## LUMBAR SPINE EXAMINATION

Alignment: normal
Inspection: unremarkable
Tenderness to palpation: L4–5, L5–S1, on both sides, right sciatic notch, and right sciatic nerve.
Muscle spasm: severe and on both sides
Range of motion: decreased 50 percent and painful
Skin: unremarkable

## SPINE EXAMINATION

Nerve provocation: Right straight-leg raising was positive at thirty degrees. Left straight-leg raising was negative. Contralateral straight-leg raising was negative. Right and left femoral nerve stress testing were negative.

## LOWER EXTREMITIES EXAMINATION

Examination of the lower extremities was basically unremarkable.

## VASCULAR EXAMINATION

Unremarkable with symmetric and normal pulses, color, and warmth.

## NEUROLOGICAL EXAMINATION

Motor, sensation, and deep tendon reflexes were normal. Babinski response is negative bilaterally. Clonus is negative bilaterally.

Long tract findings: negative bilaterally

## OFFICE X-RAYS

The following routine roentgenograms were taken today and reviewed with the patient.

Lumbar anteroposterior and lateral.
Findings: degenerative disk disease L4–5 and L5–S1
Alignment: normal
Bone density: normal
Sacroiliac joints: normal
Sacrum and coccyx: normal
Hip joints: unremarkable

## PROVISIONAL DIAGNOSIS

Lumbar spine: herniated nucleus pulposus (ICD-9-CM: 722.10)

## RECOMMENDATIONS—TESTS

Lumbar MRI.

## RECOMMENDATIONS—TREATMENT

A total of twenty sessions of sixty minutes' manual therapy is recommended for twice a week for ten weeks. Each treatment consists of fifteen minutes of interview to gather updates regarding the client symptoms and thirty minutes of hands-on treatment time, consisting of deep tissue, myofascial release, and neuromuscular therapy. The remaining time is used to assess range of motion and pain levels.

## RECOMMENDATIONS—MEDICATIONS

None.

## RECOMMENDATIONS—SURGERY

None.

## RECOMMENDATIONS—WORK

No return to work at this time.

## COUNSELING

The diagnosis, prognosis, treatment options, risks, and alternatives were discussed in detail using language understandable to this particular patient. The interpretation of the tests delineated above has been discussed with the patient in appropriate detail to his/her satisfaction. Conservative instructions and restrictions have been reviewed with the patient and have been understood. Questions have been elicited, and all questions have been answered to the patient's satisfaction in understandable terms.

## FOLLOW-UP PLAN

The patient was scheduled for a follow-up office appointment after the above testing is completed. He was instructed to contact me in the interval for any neurologic problems or worsening condition.

## DISCLOSURE

I declare under penalty of perjury that the information contained in this report and its attachments, if any, is true and correct to the best of my knowledge and belief.

_____
DR. NAEEM SHARIEFF
*Acupressure Specialist*

## Vet Pain Care

8836 Saddle Street, West Hills, CA 91307　　　　Tel: (818) 000-1234

---

| | |
|---|---|
| Horse Name: | Champ |
| Date of visit: | 11/01/2011 |
| Time of visit: | 2:30 PM |
| Examination: | Equine Injury |
| Owner Name: | Eddie Murphy Jr. |
| Owner Address: | 7018 Roscoe Blvd., Reseda, CA 91335 |
| Owner Phone: | (818) 011- 2345 |
| Veterinarian: | Kathleen Johnson |
| Check Mark: | ☐ Vet Consulted ☐ Report sent to Vet |
| Today's Date: | 12/26/2011 |

## EQUINE MASSAGE THERAPY REPORT

### HISTORY OF INJURY

The horse is thirteen years old, black gelding quarter horse/thoroughbred living in Porter Ranch with his owner, who requested massage therapy for his horse who fell while loping in the farm. Champ hit his head and took a major impact on his left front carpus. His carpus was swollen for a week and healed after veterinary examination.

### CHIEF COMPLAINT

<u>Left side of the horse</u>
Serratus ventralis (cervical portion) was very tight.
Trapezius (cervical portion) had a knot.
Subclavius (anterior deep pectoral) had knots.
Triceps brachii was very tight.
Anterior superficial (descending) pectoral
Biceps brachialis
Extensor carpi radialis

Common digital extensor
Lateral ulnar

Right side of the horse
Serratus ventralis (cervical portion) was very tight.
Deltoid
Teres minor (deep)
Triceps brachii was very tight

## DIAGNOSIS

Shoulder and neck pain.

## MEDICATION

MSM (methyl sufonyl methane), Corta-Flx, MyoGesic-CS, and monthly injection.

## TREATMENT PLAN

Massage therapy to reduce muscle tightness in the affected area. Deep pressure was applied to improve blood circulation. The therapy helps to restore muscle tissue mobility and break down adhesions.

Cold compresses to left front carpus (knee) until swelling reduces.
Light exercise would be beneficial to improve flexibility.
No forced stretches.
A follow-up massage is scheduled after five days.

## DECLARATION

I declare that the information provided here is true and correct to the best of my knowledge and belief.

Respectfully submitted,

_____

MAHARAJA, LMT

Executed at Los Angeles, California

Enclosure: one image

# Equine Image

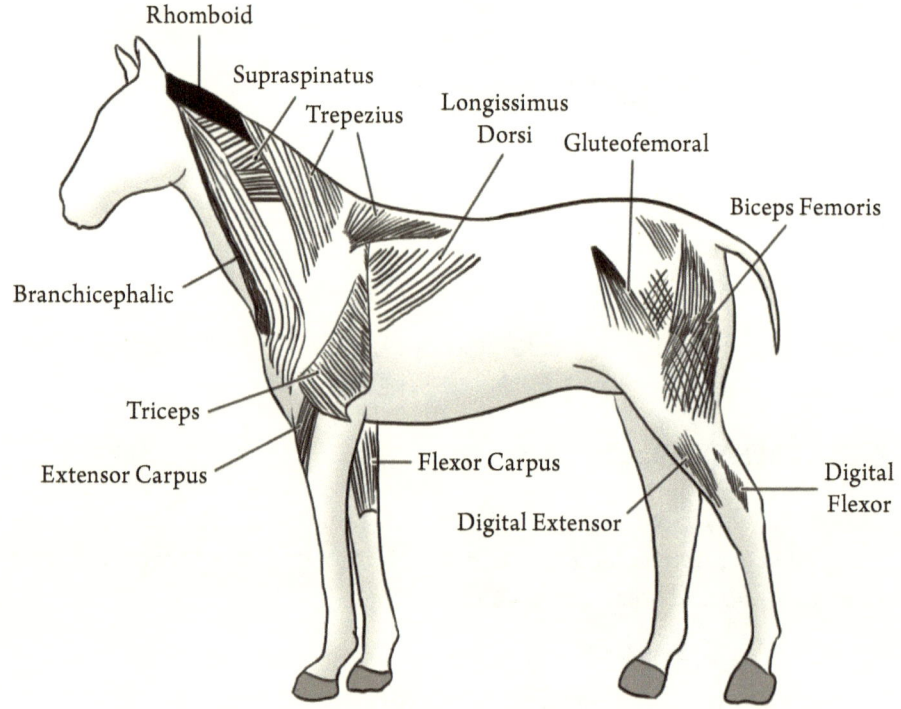

# Alien Pain Care Clinic ™

108 Welcome Street, NJ 07802                    Tel: (551) 000-0000

---

        Patient Name:     James Lee
        Employer:         Overseas Services
        Examination:      Explosion Medical Report
        Date of Loss:      08/26/10
        Claim No:         605-000055
        SSN:              xxx-xx-1234
        Today's Date:     September 29, 2010

## ACCIDENT

This patient was suffering from pain in neck, low back, bilateral knees, and dizziness due to injuries sustained when the truck was hit by a bomb while working in Iraq.

## PRESENT COMPLAINT

1. Pain on the top of his head that radiates into the posterior aspect of his neck when his head is exposed to cold weather.
2. Constant ringing in the ears.
3. Hearing loss that attributes to the accident.
4. Constant neck pain.
5. Numbness in arms, hands, fingers.
6. Discomfort in midback.
7. Constant pain in low back. The pain is worse with bending and twisting.
8. Numbness from below his waist and down both lower extremities that only occurs with prolonged sitting.
9. Bilateral hip pain that radiates down the anterior aspects of both lower extremities to the knees. The pain comes on with weight bearing and

alternates from side to side. The painful hip is better when holding the cane.
10. Eye pain, blurry vision, heartburn, dizziness, chest pain, nausea.
11. Post-traumatic stress disorder with anger, anxiety, depression, and mood swing.

## EXAMINATION CHECKLIST

1. Cervical/Neck Motion
   Right-side rotation ☐ Good ☐ Bad
   Left-side rotation ☐ Good ☐ Bad

2. Shoulder Motion
   Right-side rotation ☐ Good ☐ Bad
   Left-side rotation ☐ Good ☐ Bad

3. Straight-leg raise to 45 degrees bilaterally
   ☐ Good ☐ Bad

4. Lumbar Motion
   Side bending ☐ Good ☐ Bad
   Rotation ☐ Good ☐ Bad

5. Hip Motion
   Right ☐ Good ☐ Bad
   Left ☐ Good ☐ Bad

6. Knee Motion
   Right ☐ Good ☐ Bad
   Left ☐ Good ☐ Bad

7. Normal Reflexes ☐ Good ☐ Bad

8. Loss of strength in lower extremities

9. Diminished lower extremities sensation

## PAST ILLNESS

Patient denied major and minor surgeries.

## RECOMMENDATION

Martial arts medical massage and physical therapy are recommended for twice a week for eight weeks.

Thank you for referring this patient.

_____

REMY A. SHARIEFF, MDAM

Date: 09/29/2010

# Dubai Pain Clinic

Villa 967 Umme Kulsoom Square,　　　　　　　　Tel: (971) 1234-5678
Al Waheed Road, Dubai UAE

---

|  |  |
|--|--|
| Patient Name: | Moin Ahmed |
| Examination: | Facial Paralysis |
| Referring Physician: | Dr. Surfaraz Khan |
| Examination Date: | 10/30/11 |
| Today's Date: | 11/20/11 |

## PATIENT HISTORY

The patient is a forty-nine-year-old East Indian male, working as a construction worker in a local company, who was struck in the head by a heavy beam that fell on him from the third floor. Although he was wearing a hard hat, the impact knocked him down. He was unconscious for a while and was taken to the hospital by coworkers.

## CHIEF COMPLAINT

Right side of face paralyzed.

## DIAGNOSIS

Facial paralysis and depression.

## TREATMENT PLAN

Martial arts medical therapy three times per week for ten weeks.

**Primary acupressure points:**

| | | | |
|--|--|--|--|
| ST 1, 2, 3, 4, 5, 6, and 7 | SI 18 and 19 | SJ 21, 22 and 23 | UB 1 and 2 |
| DU 25, 26, and 27 | LI 19 and 20 | GB 1, 2, 3, 4, 5, 6, and 7 | GB 14 |
| REN 24 | | | |

**Secondary acupressure points:**

DU 16 or GV 16    DU 20 or GV 20    GB 20
Physiotherapy using warmer, hot pack, and lamp methods.

## DISCUSSION

Facial paralysis can occur for many reasons. The most common forms are as under:

1. Bell's palsy or idiopathic disease
2. Pregnancy or postchildbirth
3. Möbius syndrome
4. Ramsay Hunt syndrome
5. Guillain-Barré syndrome
6. Neurofibromatosis Type 2 (NF2)
7. Traumatic injury or accident
8. Herpes simplex virus
9. Lyme disease or Lyme borreliosis
10. Acoustic neuroma or vestibular schwannoma
11. Encephalitis
12. Mastoiditis
13. Polio
14. Tuberculosis
15. Diabetes mellitus

It is the most common form of acute paralysis of the seventh (facial) cranial nerve, affecting twenty-three of one hundred thousand people at any time. The exact cause is not known. Swelling and compression of the facial nerve may be contributing factors to this condition. Up to 80 percent of people experience spontaneous recovery. Some people suffer from complete paralysis of one side of the face, including the inability to blink while others suffer from partial paralysis. Complete recovery from partial paralysis is likely within a few months. Recovery varies more for those who seek aggressive treatment approach and dedicated to recover faster.

The kind of acupressure used to treat this patient paralysis is kung fu acupressure therapy, which has unique and distinctive characteristics without the use of electrical and mechanical device. It is purely hands-on manual therapy. The practitioner not only focuses the pressure points, but also aids in the release of the muscular tension and energy blockage, which opens the circulation of vital energy/chi.

## DECLARATION

I declare that the information provided herein is true and correct to the best of my knowledge and belief.

_____
NAEEM SHARIEFF, MDAM

Executed at Dubai, United Arab Emirates
Date: November 20, 2011

Enclosures: Images

## Images of Facial Nerve

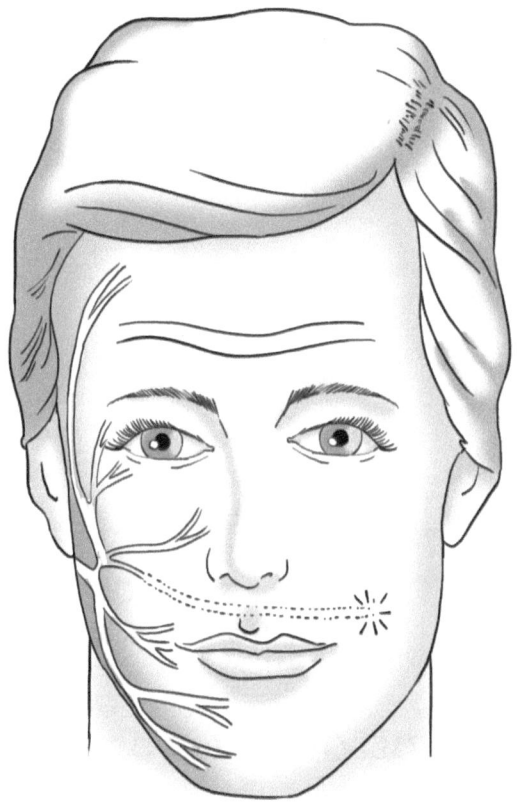

**Facial paralysis is the total loss of voluntary muscle movement of one side.**

# Sharif Pain Care Clinic ™

336 Huge Tree Street, West Hills, CA 91307      Tel: (818) 123-4567

---

November 19, 2011

Law Offices of Nobles
22711 Victory Blvd.
West Hills, CA 91307

Attention: Mr. Benikoff, Esq.

| | |
|---|---|
| Regarding: | Patrick Kumanov |
| SSN: | xxx-xx-1234 |
| Employer: | City of Hope |
| Insurance: | Jumper Insurance Services |
| Claim No: | RI 06878300-WC-011 |
| WCAB No: | VNO 0577099, ADJ 7746578 |
| Date of Injury: | 07/31/11 |

## FOLLOW-UP REPORT

The patient is returning to my attention and is still complaining of right knee pain. His physical examination is unchanged. The patient has enough medications provided by his primary treating physician. As such, no medications were ever provided in our office. I am still awaiting authorization from the insurance carrier for therapeutic sessions.

In regard to the right shoulder, the patient should continue with physiotherapy, range of motion exercises, and therapeutic modalities.

Disability status as well as permanent and stationary issues will be addressed by the primary treating physician.

I hope the above information has been helpful to you, and if I can provide you with any further information, please do not hesitate to contact my office.

I declare under penalty of perjury that I have not violated the provisions of California Labor Code 139.3 and that the contents of this report and attached billing are true and correct to the best of my knowledge. I also affirm that I have not violated any section of Labor Code 4628. Please see attached itemized billing with ICD-9 diagnosis code(s). The foregoing declaration is executed on the date of this report and signed by myself in the County of Los Angeles, California.

Thank you for your attention in this matter.

Sincerely,

_____

Naeem Sharieff, MDAM
Board Certified, Alternative Medicine
License No: 1234567

cc: Jumper Insurance Services
    PO Box 12345
    Tucson, AZ 85734

    Law Offices of Nobles
    22711 Victory Blvd.
    West Hills, CA 91307

**BILLING STATEMENT NOT ATTACHED**

# Dubai Pain Clinic

Villa 967 Umme Kulsoom Square,　　　　　　　　Tel: (971) 1 234-5678
Al Waheed Road, Dubai UAE

---

|  |  |
|---|---|
| Patient Name: | Omer Bin Abdul Aziz |
| Examination: | Headache |
| Referring Physician: | Dr. Surfaraz Khan |
| Examination Date: | 10/31/11 |
| Today's Date: | 11/11/11 |

## PATIENT HISTORY

The patient is a forty-nine-year-old Middle Eastern male working as a computer programmer in a local newspaper and required to do ten to fifteen hours overtime per week.

## CHIEF COMPLAINT

Left-side headache radiating to the temple area.

## VITAL SIGN

Blood Pressure: 125/60
Pain Level:     9/10
Pulse Left:     Weak
Pulse Right:    Wiry thread

## DIAGNOSIS

Headache, reddish and painful eyes.

## MEDICATION

The patient is taking aspirin and Tylenol as pain medication.

## TREATMENT PLAN

Acupressure therapy to relieve headache and eye pain.

Primary Pressure Points: LI 4, LV 3, GB 20, GV 16, GV 20

Secondary Pressure Points: GB 04 to GB 19, GV15 to GV24, TW 22 and 23, ST 08

First treatment of thirty minutes helps to reduce pain level from 9/10 to 6/10.

The patient is schedule for three times per week for two weeks.

This treatment not only helps to reduce pain level, but also clears the mind and benefits the brain.

## DISCUSSION

There is a wide variety of acupressure styles, such as jin shin, shiatsu, su jok, tuina, atmena, and reflexology. The kind of acupressure used to treat this patient headache and eye pain is kung fu acupressure therapy, which has unique characteristics. There is no electrical or mechanical device used to treat pain. It is purely hands-on manual therapy. The practitioner not only focuses on the pressure points but also aids the release of the muscular tension and energy blockage, which opens the circulation of chi energy.

There are five major points to treat headache: LI 4 (large intestine), LV 3 (liver), GB 20 (gallbladder), GV 16 and GV 20 (governing vessel), besides these, there are many secondary points, which are also helpful to relieve headache and eyestrain.

All that bunched-up energy in the head needs a reminder that there is plenty of space down into the torso, the arms, hands, legs, and feet. Once the energy spreads out of the head and down into the body, the chi is flowing, harmony is returned, and headache disappears.

## DECLARATION

I declare that the information provided herein is true and correct to the best of my knowledge and belief.

_____
NAEEM SHARIEFF, MDAM

Executed at Dubai, United Arab Emirates
Date: November 11, 2011

# Alien Pain Care Clinic ™

336 Huge Tree Street, West Hills, CA 91307        Tel: (818) 000 - 1234

---

Patient Name:         Saba Zlotolow
SSN:                  xxx-xx-1234
Examination:          Chronic Pain Syndrome
Referring Physician:  Dr. Surfaraz Khan
Examination Date:     09/29/2011
Today's Date:         10/31/2011

## INDEPENDENT MEDICAL EXAM

### CASE HISTORY

The patient tells me that on 09/28/11 she was the belted passenger riding in the front seat of her car, which apparently ran into the side of a delivery truck at approximately forty-five miles per hour. The patient sustained a temporary loss of consciousness. She was taken to the emergency room, where cervical spine x-rays were taken. She was given a soft cervical collar and pain medication. Then she was subsequently released.

Next day, she went to her family physician for further evaluation. Dr. Surfaraz referred the patient to our office for therapeutic evaluation and treatment.

### CHIEF COMPLAINT

Ongoing neck pain that was radiating across her upper back and shoulders. This was aggravated with prolonged sitting or standing.

### PAST HISTORY

The patient denied any previous injuries or accidents to her cervical spine prior to the motor vehicle accident on 09/28/ 2011.

## WORK HISTORY

Work history revealed that at the time of the accident, the patient was a student in a local college and was performing social work in the community.

## DIAGNOSTIC IMAGING

Review of diagnostic imaging noted that an MRI was taken for cervical spine due to ongoing neck pain. This was taken at a local hospital on 09/28/11, which was reported as an unremarkable study.

## PHYSICAL EXAMINATION

Initial evaluation of the cervical spine demonstrated that flexion was capable of 50/60 degrees. Extension was 45/50 degrees. Right lateral bending was 40/45 degrees. Left lateral bending was 45/45 degrees. Right rotation was 75/80 degrees and left rotation was 70/80 degrees. Most of her pain noted was with end range with flexion and extension. Sensory, motor, and reflex examinations were within normal limits. Compression test was positive for increasing neck pain. Distraction test was positive, whereas traction gave relief. Jackson test was positive. O'Donoghue was positive. Subluxation was detected at C4, C5, and T1. Muscle spasm was noted in the trapezius.

## TREATMENT

Treatment consisted of spinal manipulation adjunct with therapeutic modalities of acupressure, shiatsu, martial arts medical massage, myofascial release, and a home-based exercise program. As previously mentioned, she had emergency medical care and follow-up with her family physician.

## DIAGNOSIS IMPRESSION

1. Cervical spine facet syndrome
2. Subluxation to the cervical spine
3. Myofascial pain syndrome

The entire above are directly causally related to the motor vehicle accident.

## PATIENT PROGRESS

At the time of the patient's last visit with me on 10/28/11, she was noted improved status in regard to her initial chief complaint of cervical spine pain. Her range of motion returned to full range. She had intermittent discomfort in her cervical spine that was no longer constant. She felt she was benefitted from the treatment. She has to continue with home exercise program for physical fitness and strength and has to continue once-a-month therapeutic sessions for six months. Presently, she has a mild upper-extremity pain or complaint at this time.

## PROGNOSIS

The patient's overall prognosis appeared to be good with the treatment plan, which consisted of acupressure therapy and rehabilitation over a six-month period. With such, her prognosis may have been fair. Overall, in my opinion, the patient sustained a temporary disabling condition, not allowing her to perform usual and all normal activities of daily living at her regular capacity because of her motor vehicle accident. She continued to go through school yet was attending with pain. In my opinion, if she was in the workforce with a moderate to heavy job-classification demand, she would have been classified as being totally disabled for approximately a four-month time, where at the juncture she was under regular active and aggressive care in this office. Nonetheless, because of the traumatic impact she was involved in, the likelihood of future posttraumatic degenerative changes in her involved joints would certainly be considered a significant one. She has to continue home spinal exercises for strength and resistance.

## DECLARATION

I declare that the information provided herein is true and correct to the best of my knowledge and belief.

Respectfully submitted,

---

FARAH WASEEM
*Oriental Medical Doctor*

# NAEEM SHARIEFF, BA, LLB, MA, MDAM
*Acupressure Specialist*
1947 Roswell Street, Suite 100
Los Angeles, CA 91335
Tel: (818) 000-0000

September 29, 2011

Staff Compensation Insurance Fund
PO Box 19262
Los Angeles, CA 90009

Attention: Ms. Joana Bridge, Claim Adjuster

| | |
|---|---|
| Regarding: | Jose Cruz |
| Occupation: | Plumber |
| Employer: | Bigram Dixon |
| Date of Injury: | 05/21/11 |
| Claim Number: | DJ 149628 |
| Our Record: | RN 9948 |

## INITIAL ACUPRESSURE REPORT

Dear Ms. Bridge,

***Introduction:***

Mr. Jose Cruz, a thirty-year-old male, was seen at my Los Angeles office located at the above-mentioned address and examined personally by me today. This acupressure *medical evaluation* was performed at your request for the purpose of obtaining my opinion as an acupressure specialist regarding an injury claim arising out of Mr. Cruz's employment with Bigram Dixon.

This *evaluation* was conducted with the assistance of a Spanish-speaking interpreter, Carlos De La Torre, of Brilliant Translating Services. The following is a summary of this patient's current status and findings:

**SITE OF COMPLAINT**

Neck and back.

**HISTORY OF PRESENT INJURY**
(as related by the patient)

He said he had an injury but did not remember the date. I asked him to try to put it into some perspective: was it months ago, more than ten years ago, more than five years ago, six hours ago, etc. May 21, 2011 is when he happened to make a claim. He felt a dull pain in his lower back when carrying a toolbox from one floor to another sometime last year (i.e., in the year 2010). He never reported this pain. He felt fine at that time. He continued working at his usual and customary occupation, which entails doing heavy lifting and assembling boilers, so there is lifting, bending, using his hands, pushing, pulling, climbing, standing, and walking involved with the job. He has worked for this company for a whole year, and before that, he worked for a similar company for seven years. He denies having any other injuries with the other company as far as his neck and back are concerned. I asked him about other specific injuries, such as automobile accidents, slips and falls in supermarkets, drugstores, or in friends' apartments—he denies having these.

**CURRENT COMPLAINTS**

He has residual complaints at this time, he now feels fine and totally asymptomatic.

**OCCUPATIONAL TITLE AND DESCRIPTION**

This has been discussed above.

**PAST MEDICAL HISTORY**

His general health apart from the above has been good on systematic inquiry.

He just happened to go and see a shiatsupractor earlier this year. The shiatsupractor informed him that this could be industrial injury. The shiatsupractor is now giving him therapy for his complaint.

He does the same type of work that he has been doing despite having the shiatsu therapy (i.e., he is on no light duty). He feels much better after being treated by the shiatsupractor.

## PHYSICAL EXAMINATION

Physical examination shows a man of stated age in no acute distress, free of anemia, jaundice, arthritis, gouty tophi, or abnormal rashes. He walks without stick or support. He can stand on his toes and heels. His physical examination is entirely normal with a normal full range of neck and back motion carried out with alacrity; full shoulder, elbow, wrist, and finger motion; hip, knee, and ankle motion. Equal leg lengths. Normal straight-leg raising beyond ninety degrees.

Motor power, including resisted abduction, flexion, and extension of the shoulders; resisted elbow flexion and extension; grip, pinch, grasp, and release are normal and equal bilaterally. There is a lack of scapular winging.

Motor power in the extensor hallucis longus, anterior and posterior tibias, quadriceps and triceps sure is equal and intact bilaterally.

Reflexes are brisk, present, and equal at the biceps, triceps, and brachioradialis sites at both knees and both ankle. Babinski is negative. Sensation is intact throughout the dermatomes of both upper and lower extremities. There is no spasm, guarding, or tenderness in the neck muscles or in the back muscles.

Range of motion of the neck carried out actively and voluntarily by the patient, which is as follows in degrees:

|  | **Examined** | **Normal** |
|---|---|---|
| Flexion | 60 | 60 (chin to chest) |
| Extension | 40 | 40 |
| Lateral Flexion | 45/45 | 45/45 |
| Rotation | 85/85 | 85/85 |

Range of motion of the upper extremities is as follows in degrees:

| **Shoulder** | **Right** | **Left** | **Normal** |
|---|---|---|---|
| Extension | 60 | 60 | 60 |
| Abduction | 180 | 180 | 180 |
| Flexion | 180 | 180 | 180 |
| External Rotation | 90 | 90 | 90 |
| Internal Rotation | 70 | 70 | 70 |

Can touch hand to back bilaterally.

| **Elbow** | **Right** | **Left** | **Normal** |
|---|---|---|---|
| Extension | 0 | 0 | 0 |
| Flexion | 135 | 135 | 135 |

| **Forearm** | **Right** | **Left** | **Normal** |
|---|---|---|---|
| Pronation | 75 | 75 | 75 |
| Supination | 90 | 90 | 90 |

| **Wrist** | **Right** | **Left** | **Normal** |
|---|---|---|---|
| Extension | 65 | 65 | 65 |
| Flexion | 70 | 70 | 70 |
| Ulnar Deviation | 40 | 40 | 40 |
| Radial Deviation | 20 | 20 | 20 |
| Palmar Flexion | 80 | 80 | 80 |
| Dorsiflexion | 80 | 80 | 80 |

| **Thumb** | **Right** | **Left** | **Normal** |
|---|---|---|---|
| Abduction | 55 | 55 | 55 |
| Adduction | 0 | 0 | 0 |

Range of motion of the back carried out actively and voluntarily is as follows in degrees:

| | **Examined** | **Normal** |
|---|---|---|
| Flexion | 90 | 90 |
| Extension | 40 | 40 |
| Lateral Flexion | 45/45 | 45/45 |
| Rotation | 85/85 | 85/85 |

Range of motion of the joints of the lower extremities is as follows in degrees:

| Hip | Right | Left | Normal |
|---|---|---|---|
| Flexion | 120 | 120 | 120 |
| Extension | 0 | 0 | 0 |
| Internal Rotation | 45 | 45 | 45 |
| External Rotation | 45 | 45 | 45 |
| Abduction | 45 | 45 | 45 |
| Adduction | 35 | 35 | 35 |

| Knee | Right | Left | Normal |
|---|---|---|---|
| Extension | 0 | 0 | 0 |
| Flexion | 160 | 160 | 160 |

| Ankle | Right | Left | Normal |
|---|---|---|---|
| Dorsiflexion (Extension) | 35 | 35 | 35 |
| Plantar Flexion (Flexion) | 50 | 50 | 50 |

| Foot | Right | Left | Normal |
|---|---|---|---|
| Inversion | 35 | 35 | 35 |
| Eversion | 20 | 20 | 20 |

| Great Toe Metatarsophalangeal Joint | Right | Left | Normal |
|---|---|---|---|
| Flexion | 35 | 35 | 35 |
| Extension | 60 | 60 | 60 |

## REVIEW OF OUTSIDE MEDICAL RECORDS

There is a report by a shiatsupractor, namely, Maria Arriola, on April 18, 2009.

## DIAGNOSIS

Normal acupressure examination.

## DISCUSSION

It is rather a stretch of the imagination to believe that there is any connection between a long-forgotten minor ache that he had in his back sometime last year with a need for shiatsu therapy on an industrial basis a year later in a patient or person that can do his job without any difficulty and currently has no symptoms whatsoever and has a normal acupressure examination. There was never any industrial specific injury that required treatment or caused disability, nor is there any right now, nor is there any need for any continuing shiatsu therapy on an industrial basis. He has no subjective or objective findings of any disability.

Should there be any further inquiries regarding the above-named patient, I would be happy to try and answer them.

## DISCLOSURE

The history, physical examination review of medical records, and dictation of this report were performed by myself (the report was typed by a professional transcriptionist). The opinions expressed herein are exclusively my own.

## DECLARATION

I declare that the information provided here is true and correct to the best of my knowledge and belief and nothing has been concealed.

Furthermore, I appreciate the opportunity to participate in the evaluation and treatment of this patient. Please call me should you have any further questions or if this office can be of further assistance.

_____

DR. NAEEM SHARIEFF
*Acupressure Specialist*

Executed at Los Angeles, California
Date: September 29, 2011

# Taxila Pain Clinic

336 Harris Hill Road,   Tel: (201) 000 - 1234
Williamsville, Buffalo, NY 91441

---

Patient Name:        Mawla Buksh
SSN:                 xxx-xx-1234
Examination:         Jaw Pain
Referring Physician: Dr. Surfaraz Khan
Examination Date:    10/30/2011
Today's Date:        10/31/2011

## CHIEF COMPLAINT

Jaw pain.

## PATIENT HISTORY

The patient is a thirty-eight-year-old male who started out having toothache in the left lower side of the mouth and that is now radiating into the jaw and toward his left ear.

## CLINICAL EXAMINATION

The patient looked well and was very cooperative.

VITAL SIGNS: Temperature is 98.2; blood pressure is 168/84; pulse is 87; respirations, 16; oxygen saturation is 100 percent on room air and interpreted as normal.

CONSTITUTIONAL: No fever or chills, no fatigue or weakness.

HEENT: No headache. No neck pain. No eye pain or vision change. No rhinorrhea. No sinus congestion, pressure, or pain. No sore throat. No throat swelling. No ear pain or hearing change. No pressure in the ears. No sign of ear infection.

MOUTH: The gums are normal, without any erythema, swelling, or evidence of infection.

NECK: Full range of motion.

CARDIOVASCULAR: Heart is in regular rate and rhythm without murmur, rub, or gallop. No chest pain.

RESPIRATIONS: No shortness of breath.

GASTROINTESTINAL: No nausea or vomiting. No abdominal pain.

MUSCULOSKELETAL: No abnormalities were noted on the back, arms, or legs. The patient has normal use of the extremities.

SKIN: No rashes or lesions.

NEUROLOGIC: No vision or hearing loss. No speech change.

PSYCHIATRIC: The patient is alert and oriented. Normal mood. No evidence of clinical intoxication.

**PAST MEDICAL HISTORY**

None

**PAST SURGICAL HISTORY**

None

**CURRENT MEDICATIONS**

None

## ALLERGIES

None

## SOCIAL HISTORY

The patient smokes marijuana but does not smoke cigarettes.

## DIAGNOSES

1. Acute left jaw pain
2. Elevated blood pressure

## TREATMENT PLAN

Sixty minutes of acupressure therapy is needed twice a week for four weeks to relieve pain.

Surgery not needed.

## DECLARATION

I declare that the information provided herein is true and correct to the best of my knowledge and belief.

_____

IBRAHIM W. SHARIEFF
*Acupressure Specialist*

Executed at Buffalo, New York
Date: October 31, 2011

Enclosure: one image

# Image for Treatment

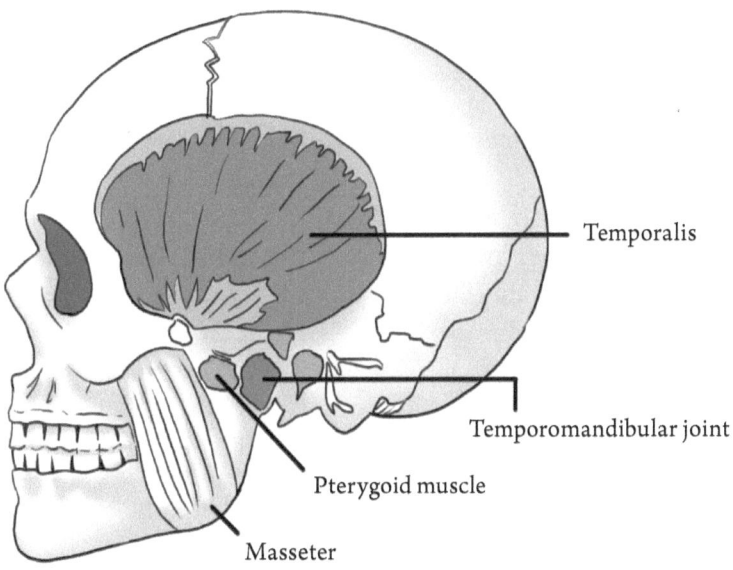

**Focusing on masseter muscle only to relieve pain**

# Alien Pain Care Clinic ™

336 Huge Tree Street, West Hills, CA 91307          Tel: (818) 000-1234

---

Patient Name:        Asim Durrani
SSN:                 xxx-xx-1234
Examination:         Left Knee
Referring Physician: Dr. Mehnaz Khan
Examination Date:    10/01/2011
Today's Date:        10/22/2011

## JOB DESCRIPTION

The patient is a forty-eight-year-old Iranian male who worked as an aircraft mechanic for Royal Airlines for the last ten years. Presently, he is on disability due to increased pain.

## CHIEF COMPLAINT

Left knee pain.

## HISTORY OF INJURY

Mr. Asim Durrani reports that he was working on an aircraft when he fell between the airplane and a stand with about an eighteen-inch gap in between. He injured his left knee and underwent two arthroscopic procedures followed by patellar replacement and subsequently a total left knee arthroplasty on July 03, 2011.

The patient reports that he has undergone a full course of physical therapy and complains primarily of pain in the anterior aspect of the left knee and primarily over the medial and lateral tibial components with pain extending proximally to the distal femur and distally down into the anterior tibial plateau area. He has intermittent numbness and tingling in the posterolateral thigh.

His pain is worse with walking and is associated with swelling, popping, and grinding. He complains of pins-and-needles sensation over the area of the common peroneal nerve overlying the fibular head.

The patient underwent a left-knee MRI in September of 2011 revealing nonspecific edema anterior to the patellar tendon but no evidence of an acute fracture or a patellofemoral ligament avulsion or abnormality.

He has continued to complain of persistent instability and pain. His pain is described as constant, shooting, cramping, aching, throbbing, pulling, sharp, and stabbing in nature. It occasionally awakens him at night. He does relate that he gained weight since his injury.

Dr. Haqqani recommended him for physical therapy. The patient continues at home with quadriceps and hamstrings exercises. He has discontinued use of his knee brace and would like to avoid surgery, if at all possible.

## MEDICATIONS

No medications.

## ALLERGIES

Morphine, Bactrim, and Benadryl.

## FAMILY HISTORY

Remarkable for cervical cancer, heart disease, and diabetes.

## SOCIAL HISTORY

The patient is not working. Rates his stress level as an 8/10. He is divorced with no children. Does not smoke, drink, or utilize illicit substances.

## REVIEW OF SYSTEMS

A thirteen-point review of systems was surveyed including constitutional, HEENT, cardiac, pulmonary, gastrointestinal, endocrine, integumentary, hematological, immunological, neurological, musculoskeletal, psychological, and rheumatological. Review of systems is negative.

## PHYSICAL EXAMINATION

Weight, 220 pounds; temperature, 97.6; pulse, 74; blood pressure 140/94. The patient walks with an antalgic gait to the left. He has pain vocalization with standing, walking, and range of motion of the knee.

The skin is warm and dry to the touch with peripheral pulses equally palpable over the radial, dorsalis pedis, and posterior tibial areas.

There is sensitivity over the distal aspect of his midline scar. There is edema over the anterior tibial plateau and tenderness over both the medial, as well as lateral aspects of the tibial plateau. There is no discoloration. No trophic changes. He is able to perform a straight leg lift and has otherwise normal engagement of all his distal musculature.

## DIAGNOSIS IMPRESSION

Status post–left knee injury with subsequent knee replacement and continued chronic pain on the left knee. He may have patellofemoral and/or tibial plateau–related pain as well.

## TREATMENT PLAN

I have scheduled him for a chronic pain program in our clinic. The first appointment is scheduled on October 25, 2011 at 4:00 PM for one-hour acupressure therapy.

## DECLARATION

I declare that the information provided herein is true and correct to the best of my knowledge and belief.

_____
SHOAIB SALEEM, OMD

Executed at Los Angeles, California
Date: October 22, 2011

# Alien Pain Care Clinic ™

336 Huge Tree Street, West Hills, CA 91307　　　Tel: (818) 000 - 1234

---

|  |  |
|---|---|
| Patient Name: | Kali Devi |
| SSN: | xxx-xx-1234 |
| Examination: | Left-Side Paralysis |
| Examination Date: | 09/05/2011 |
| Today's Date: | 12/05/2011 |

Manual therapy for paralysis.

## CLINICAL HISTORY

Kali Devi, a sixty-year-old Indian female, had a sudden stroke of paralysis on the left side of her body. The affected area was cold, and there was a marked footdrop. She was completely bedridden and had to be physically carried to the restroom. Her family brought her to this clinic for treatment.

## DIAGNOSIS IMPRESSION

Left-side paralysis

## METHOD APPLIED

North pole under the palm of the left hand and south pole under the sole of the left foot

## TREATMENT PLAN

1. Three thousand gauss of high-powered magnets was used in this treatment, which has a capacity to lift 10 kg of iron weight.

2. The duration of application of magnets was ten minutes initially, which was gradually increased to fifteen minutes twice daily.
3. Mixed magnetized water (north pole and south pole) was given three times a day.
4. This water was prepared on top of a 3,000 G power magnet for eight hours.
5. Dosage was 2 oz., or 50 mL, each time, before breakfast and after big meal.
6. South pole–magnetized oil was used externally. Before the application of magnet.
7. This oil was prepared in direct sunlight for twenty-one days in blue bottle on the top of a 3,000 G power south pole magnet.
8. Physiotherapy on daily basis.
9. Sunbathing fifteen to twenty minutes daily between the hours of 7:00 AM to 11:00 AM.
10. Full-body deep tissue massage was given twice a week for an hour.

## RESULTS

After three months of treatment, she was able to sit and move to the kitchen and bathroom by herself with the help of a walking stick. The left arm is still slightly cold and circulation has clearly improved at the left forearm. Sitting, she can extend the left leg horizontally and succeeds in raising her arm almost to shoulder height. I believe that it takes another three months for full recovery.

## DECLARATION

I declare that the information provided herein is true and correct to the best of my knowledge and belief.

_____

SURFARAZ KHAN, MDAM

Enclosure(s): Two images of magneto therapy

# Images of Magneto Therapy

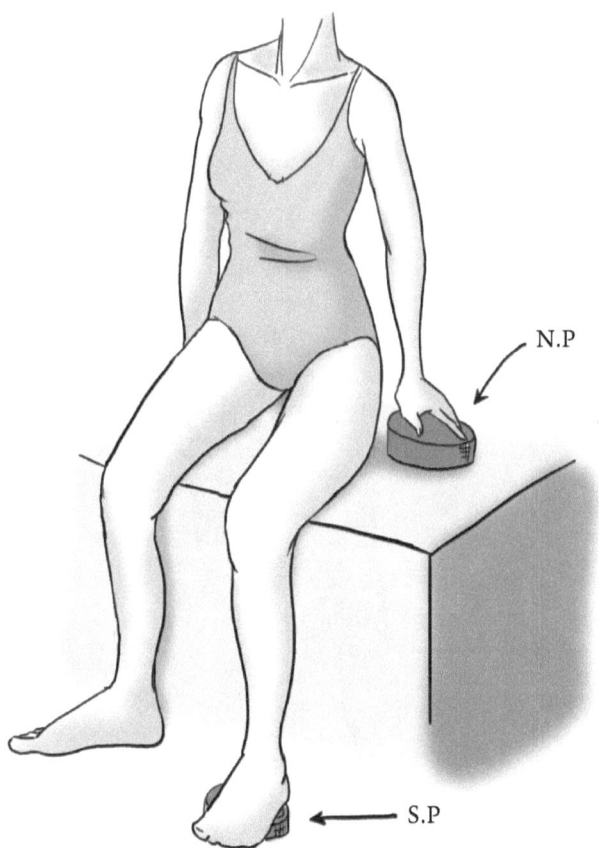

**Figure 1**

# Images of Magneto Therapy

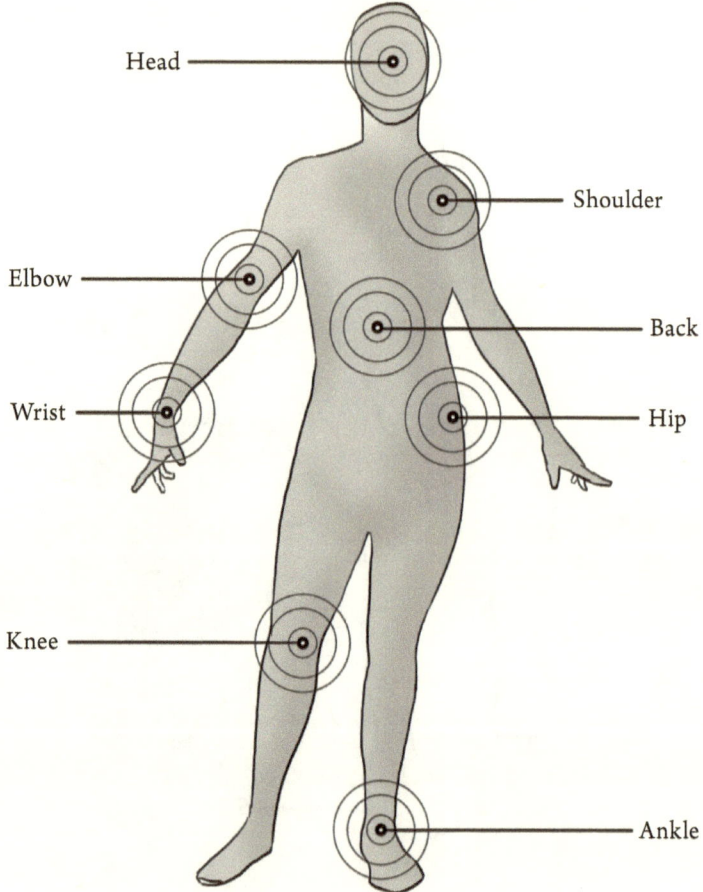

**Circles indicate blood circulation.
Figure 2**

# Alien Pain Care Clinic ™

336 Huge Tree Street, West Hills, CA 91307          Tel: (818) 000-1234

                Patient Name:         Sara Aziz
                SSN:                  xxx-xx-1234
                Examination:          Left Wrist
                Referring Physician:  Dr. Mehnaz Khan
                Examination Date:     10/01/2011
                Today's Date:         10/22/2011

## JOB DESCRIPTION

The patient is a thirty-nine-year-old Indian female who has worked as an administrative assistant in an advertising firm for the last eight years. Presently, she is on medical leave due to increased pain.

## CHIEF COMPLAINT

Left wrist pain with edema and swelling in the ulnar styloid region.

## HISTORY OF INJURY

The patient has a previous history of a traumatic left-wrist injury, which has left her with a chronic scapholunate problem and possibly other problems in her wrist. However, she was doing relatively fine and tolerating the wrist soreness that she had, which is day to day, but it has not gotten much worse until this injury. Once she lifted the object out of the back of her chair and it started to hurt, then she was significantly more affected than she had been before, and now, pain is more on the ulnar side of her wrist than on the radial side of her wrist. She is here now for evaluation.

## CLINICAL EXAMINATION

Musculoskeletal: The patient has point tenderness to palpation along the ulnar-styloid extensor carpi ulnaris tendon with some minor tenderness at the triangular fibrocartilage complex region, as well as the lunotriquetral joint. There is some minor soreness, but not nearly as sore at the scapholunate ligament with dorsiflexion, thirty degrees; palmar flexion, thirty degrees; radial deviation, five degrees; and ulnar deviation, zero degrees. Supination/pronation grossly intact without significant signs of instability.

Skin: No skin breakdown or hyperhidrosis.
Neurologic: Negative signs of compressive median nerve neuropathy.
Vascular: Intact

## RADIOLOGICAL EXAM

X-rays, three views of the wrist of good penetrance and quality, reveal scapholunate widening of a slack wrist with a possible ulnar-styloid nonunion, with a possible occult distal radius fracture fibrous union. MRI report reviewed.

## RESTRICTIONS

This patient requires work restrictions. This should take the form of repetitive hand use and over-the-shoulder-level activities. This patient should also not lift more than five pounds.

## MEDICAL TREATMENT

In consideration of the persistent symptomatology, this patient requires additional evaluation by way of MRI/MRA by a radiologist. This will assist in clarifying the pathomechanical basis of her continued symptomatology and limitations with respect to activities of daily living.

Furthermore, acupressure therapy may help her relief from chronic pain and discomfort twice a week for ten weeks.

## DECLARATION

I declare that the information provided herein is true and correct to the best of my knowledge and belief.

_____

DR. NAEEM SHARIEFF
*Acupressure Specialist*

Executed at Los Angeles, California
Date: October 22, 2011

Enclosure: One image

# Injured body part image—carpus

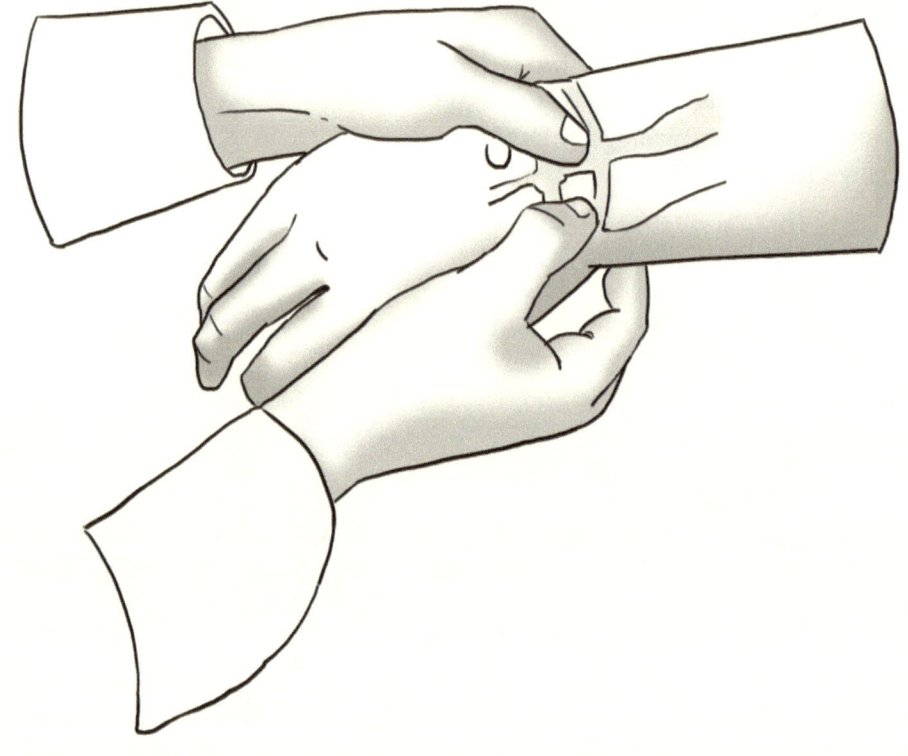

## East Coast Back Pain Clinic

333 Grand Trunk Road  
Williamsville, Buffalo, NY 91441

Tel: (201) 000-1234  
Fax: (201) 000-1235

---

| | |
|---|---|
| Patient Name: | Mayra Lee |
| SSN: | xxx-xx-1234 |
| Examination: | Low-Back Pain |
| Referring Physician: | Dr. Surfaraz Khan |
| Examination Date: | 06/07/2011 |
| Today's Date: | 07/24/2011 |

## JOB DESCRIPTION

The patient is a forty-seven-year-old Hispanic female working as an administrative assistant for the City of Gold in the last five years and sustained a work-related injury on 06/01/2011.

## HISTORY OF INJURY

The patient bent over to put a piece of paper in a file at her office and got severe low-back pain radiating to her left lower extremity. She was taken by ambulance to the hospital for treatment. X-rays were taken, and she was told that her bones were okay, and she was given a muscle relaxant and sent to Occupational Medicine, where she was prescribed Naprosyn.

The patient stated that in the interval of time after being seen at the hospital, she became progressively worse to the point where the low-back pain was inducing severe headaches. She stated that the pain was substantially handicapping with respect to any activities of daily living. She was having substantial difficulty in sleeping, and when she rolled over, she had sharp paroxysms of pain. The patient stated that any movement of her trunk or legs would induce a sharp increase in pain.

## DOCTOR'S FIRST REPORT OF OCCUPATIONAL INJURY

The patient was first seen by Dr. Khan on 06/01/2011 through her final examination on 06/07/2011. As of 06/07/2011, she was deemed permanent and stationary and was diagnosed of fibromyalgia syndrome. Dr. Khan continued treatment due to her medical condition.

## DIAGNOSIS IMPRESSION

Mechanical low-back pain syndrome associated with and complicated by instability at the lumbosacral junction associated with bilateral right greater than left sciatic radiculopathy.

Mechanical, thoracic, and cervical pain syndrome secondary to the stooped/antalgic posture of the lumbar spine.

Fibromyalgia syndrome.

## OBJECTIVE FINDINGS

This patient has loss of lumbar range of motion (ROM), 50 percent of extension range of motion and approximately 20 percent of flexion range of motion. Additionally, she has multiple painful myofascial trigger points, satisfying the diagnosis of fibromyalgia syndrome. These trigger points are disturbed in her lower extremities, buttocks, truncal musculature, shoulders, forearms, and neck.

## FUTURE MEDICAL TREATMENT

This patient requires the availability of treatment in the future. This will most likely consist of episodic acupuncture and/or physical therapy procedures and modalities. This patient also requires the availability of low-tech home-exercise equipment such as an exercise ball and/or exercise tubing. This patient's clinical condition encompasses discography and loss-of-motion segment integrity, and as a result, surgical intervention at a point in the future may be necessary, although it is probably not likely given an adequate response and outcome from nonsurgical interventions. This patient also requires the availability of prescription and nonprescription medications so as to control pain and/or inflammation or muscle spasm. This patient may need periods of temporary disability in the future as a result of exacerbated pain levels.

## DECLARATION

I declare that the information provided here is true and correct to the best of my knowledge and belief and nothing has been concealed.

Thank you for referring this patient.

_____

DR. REMY A. SHARIEFF

Executed at Buffalo, New York

# East Coast Back Pain Clinic

333 Grand Trunk Road  
Williamsville, Buffalo, NY 91441

Tel: (201) 000-1234  
Fax: (201) 000-1235

---

Patient Name: Sheila Petroman  
SSN: xxx-xx-1234  
Examination: Lumbar Spine  
Referring Physician: Dr. Waseem Sharieff  
Examination Date: 06/13/2011  
Today's Date: 07/24/2011

Manual therapy for pain control.

## CLINICAL HISTORY

Lower back pain. R/O disk herniation.

## TECHNIQUE

Martial arts medical massage was performed in chronic pain with the use of elbow, fingers, fist, and knuckles. The following methods were not used in this therapy: no electrical devices, no mechanical devices, no traction, no needles, no medications, no heat pad, no cold pad, no cupping, no heat lamp, no rollers and balls, no stones, no magnets, no laser, no ultrasound, no oil or lotion.

## FINDINGS

There is no abnormality noted or discovered.

## IMPRESSION

Mild disk bulging.

## RECOMMENDATION

Additional testing may be helpful, if clinically desirable and appropriate, such as magnetic resonance imaging (MRI) and a home-based exercise program consisting of stretching, strengthening, and range of motion exercises. A class of yoga or tai chi is highly recommended for faster rehabilitation.

Thank you for referring this patient.

_____
AULINE ARROBANG, LMT

# Alien Pain Care Clinic ™

336 Huge Tree Street, West Hills, CA 91307  Tel: (818) 000-1234

---

        Patient Name:           Rina Royal
        SSN:                          xxx-xx-1234
        Examination:           Multiple Injuries
        Referring Physician:   Dr. Khan
        Examination Date:     04/07/2006
        Today's Date:           06/22/2006

## HISTORY OF INJURY

The applicant was involved in a work-related accident while inside an elevator, which malfunctioned, shook, and rumbled. She pushed the button, and the elevator went to first floor, dropped, and then shot up to the fourth floor. She held on to the railing with her right arm. Her neck jolted, and she hurt her right shoulder holding on to the railing. When she got out of the elevator, she started feeling pain and stiffness in her neck. She went to her desk and reported the injury to her supervisor.

She continued work, and the pain increased radiating down her right and left arms. She stayed working, and within a week, the pains got worse, and she went to the emergency room at Best Hills Health and Rehabilitation Center. Later, she went to Dr. Khan, who ordered an MRI of the neck, which showed a mild defused disk. She was dissatisfied and ended up changing doctors and therapists. Through her attorney, she was referred to Dr. Surfaraz Khan, who referred the patient to me for alternative treatment.

## LMT FIRST REPORT

I have been selected by the employee to be the massage therapist. This claim involves pain in back, shoulders, arms and pain/numbness in left and right hands secondary to injuries she sustained in a work-related accident when the elevator malfunctioned and dropped.

## INJURED BODY PARTS AND WORKERS COMPENSATION CODES

200—Neck
319—Arm
330—Hand
420—Back
450—Shoulders

## DIAGNOSIS IMPRESSION

1. Cervical sprain/strain
2. Lumbar sprain/strain
3. Shoulder sprain/strain

## SUBJECTIVE FINDINGS

Continued throbbing, burning pain, and swelling to neck, forearms, and wrists as well as lower back spasm. Increase in pain with repetitive use of hands, such as driving, gripping, stress, typing, lifting, and cooking. The patient stated sudden pain spasm that last for hours and days at a time. Pain level in neck and upper back is increased with stress to point of inability to continue desk type of work and has to change activities or lie down for ten minutes or so in order to decrease pain. Prolonged sitting (thirty to sixty minutes) leads to left-leg pain. Patient used Robaxin and Darvocet for pain, swelling, and spasms. Low-back and leg pains lead to difficulty to sleep. Difficulty to get out of bed secondary to low-back pain. Difficulty to stand up straight secondary to pain. It took ten seconds to ten minutes to be able to be straight.

## FUTURE MEDICAL CARE

Ms. Royal required future medical care, which may include episodic physical therapy or manual therapy, as she requires ongoing treatment and monitoring for her chronic pain and long-acting narcotic use. I do not believe she is a candidate for surgery of any kind.

## TREATMENT PLAN

Therapeutic exercises, cervical range of motion exercises, shoulder wall-walk exercises, cervical isometric exercises. Reviewed with patient activities of daily living modifications: no lifting greater than five pounds; no sitting/standing for more than fifteen minutes; change in posture frequently; no neck flexion, extension, or repetitive use of upper extremity for greater than fifteen minutes per hour.

## DECLARATION

I declare that the information provided here is true and correct to the best of my knowledge and belief and nothing has been concealed.

Thank you for referring this patient.

_____

REMY A. SHARIEFF, LMT, MDAM

Executed at Los Angeles, California

# Alien Pain Care Clinic ™

336 Huge Tree Street, West Hills, CA 91307         Tel: (818) 000-1234

|                      |                    |
|----------------------|--------------------|
| Patient Name:        | Jose Cruz          |
| SSN:                 | xxx-xx-1234        |
| Examination:         | Neck Pain          |
| Referring Physician: | Dr. Surfaraz Khan  |
| Examination Date:    | 04/07/2006         |
| Today's Date:        | 06/22/2006         |

## HISTORY OF INJURY

The patient was involved in a motor vehicle accident on April 07, 2006. He stated in his report that he was on Alameda Avenue on ramp transitioning to Interstate 5, southbound around 09:15 a.m. when he was rear-ended by a Honda Accord. Mr. Cruz was driving Hyundai Sonata, which had rear-end damage, but the damage to the Honda Accord was more extensive. At the time of accident, there were no police at the scene, and his vehicle was drivable and had not been towed. He stated that he hit his head hard into the headrest, which caused him instant neck pain and pain extending up to the back of his head as well as down over his shoulder blades. He stated that the pain induced a feeling of weakness into his arms, especially by the end of the day. He stated that he would get shooting pain from his neck to his head with certain ranges of motion of his neck.

Additionally, certain ranges of motion of his neck would also cause sharp, sudden shocks of pain, which extended from his neck to his scapular areas and upper back. He stated that he has had significant difficulty in sleeping because of neck and upper back pain. He stated that it was hard to find a comfortable position so as to be able to fall asleep, and once asleep, he would reawaken several times per night as a result of pain. He stated that at times it was difficult for him to use his arms or elevate his arms as a result of the pain. Typically, the pain was worse in his left arm than in his right arm, and he experienced more episodes of the shooting pain in his left arm than right. He stated that Tylenol led to a slight reduction of pain. He stated that in general he has experienced significant handicap as result of the pain induced by the injuries he sustained in the motor vehicle accident of 04/07/06.

## PHYSICAL EXAMINATION

The physical examination was directed to pursuing the presenting symptomatology.

## IMAGING STUDIES

The findings of x-rays of the cervical spine and thoracic spine are as follows:

Overall right lateral lean of the upper thoracic spine consistent with muscle spasm/splinting. No evidence of acute osseous trauma in the thoracic spine, and the soft tissue densities are within normal limits. There was substantial rotational subluxation of C2 relative to C1.

The cervical spine demonstrates no significant degenerative changes, and the disk heights are well maintained throughout.

There is overall forward carriage of the head and neck and loss of any extension below the C7 level consistent with deep anterior cervical muscle spasm/splinting secondary to trauma. Additionally noted is failure of normal flexion between the occiput and C6 with flexion resulting in a flattening of the cervical lordosis without any reversal of the cervical lordosis on flexion. This is consistent with muscle spasming secondary to trauma.

## X-RAY REPORT

The x-ray failed to demonstrate loss of motion segment integrity by the angular motion methodology or by the translation methodology at C5/C6. The maximum differential on angular motion measurement is 2.5°. The maximum translation between C5 and C6 is 3 mm. Both these measurements fall below the standard established for the diagnosis of loss of motion segment integrity.

## DIAGNOSIS IMPRESSION

Posttrauma cervical and upper thoracic sprain/strain associated with cervicogenic headaches and cervical radiculopathy and mechanical neck pain syndrome, complicated by cochlear concussion and balance disorder related thereto.

## COURSE OF TREATMENT

Treatment for this patient was commenced on 04/15/06. This was following a comprehensive review with this patient of the history, the physical examination findings, the x-ray findings, the treatment plan, the prognosis, the procedures, alternatives and risks, and the anticipated time frame of treatment for this patient.

Treatment encompassed a multimodality and procedure approach, utilizing the treatment procedures elaborated on the patient treatment plan. These procedures encompassed both active and passive treatment modalities procedures for the purpose of actively rehabilitating this patient's cervical and upper thoracic spine, both from a functional and structural standpoint. Treatment was associated with a positive rehabilitative benefit. There were periodic evaluations, which were conducted over the course this patient's clinical management.

Thank you for referring this patient.

_____

KUAN PAO CHANG, OMD

# Dubai Pain Clinic

Villa 967 Umme Kulsoom Square,  Tel: (971) 1234-5678
Al Waheed Road, Dubai UAE

Patient Name: Mohammad Azizullah
Examination: Neck and Shoulder Pain
Referring Physician: Dr. Surfaraz Khan
Examination Date: 10/30/11
Today's Date: 11/12/11

## PATIENT HISTORY

The patient is a fifty-nine-year-old Middle Eastern male working as an operation manager in domestic airlines and required to do excessive work every week.

## CHIEF COMPLAINT

Right-side neck pain and stiffness in the shoulders.

## VITAL SIGN

Blood Pressure: 125/60
Pain Level: 10/10
Pulse Left: Deep wiry
Pulse Right: Wiry

## DIAGNOSIS

Neck pain and stiff shoulders.

## MEDICATION

The patient is taking Advil and Tylenol twice a day.

## TREATMENT PLAN

Acupressure therapy to relieve neck pain and shoulders' stiffness.
Primary pressure points of neck: GB 20, GV 14 or DU 14, GV 16, LI 18, B 10
Shoulder pressure points: GB 21, TW 15, SI 14, SI 15.
First treatment of thirty minutes helps to reduce pain level from 10/10 to 6/10.
The patient is schedule for three times per week for two weeks.
Neck stretches as home exercise.

## DISCUSSION

There is a wide variety of acupressure styles such as jin shin, shiatsu, su jok, tuina, atmena, and reflexology. The kind of acupressure used to treat this patient's neck pain and shoulder stiffness is kung fu acupressure therapy, which has unique and distinctive characteristics. There is no electrical or mechanical device used to treat pain. It is purely hands-on manual therapy. The practitioner not only focuses on the pressure points, but also aids the release of the muscular tension and energy blockage, which opens the circulation of chi energy.

The major points used to treat neck pain and shoulder stiffness is as under:

GB 20, GB 21, GV 14 or DU 14, DU 16, GV 16, TW 15, SI 14, SI 15, LI 18, and B 10.

## DECLARATION

I declare that the information provided herein is true and correct to the best of my knowledge and belief.

_____
NAEEM SHARIEFF, MDAM

Executed at Dubai, UAE
Date: November 12, 2011

Enclosures: Images of acu-points

## Images of Acu-Points

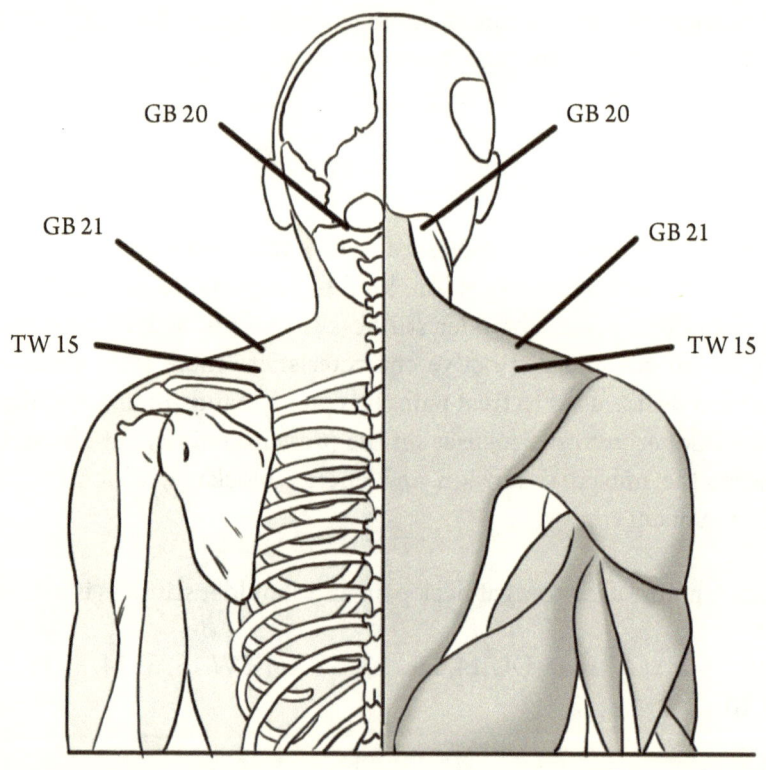

# Mumtaz Medical Center

105 Bungalow Town  Tel: (818) 000-0001
West Hills, CA 91307  Fax: (818) 000-0002

## PATIENT PROGRESS REPORT

### PATIENT INFORMATION

First Name: _____
Last Name: _____
Gender: _____
Date of Birth: _____
Date of Injury: _____
SSN/ID No: _____
WCAB Case No: _____

Street Address: _____
City: _____
State: _____ Zip Code: _____
Phone No: _____

### CLAIM ADMINISTRATOR INFORMATION

Adjuster Name: _____
Insurance Carrier: _____
Claim No: _____
Street Address: _____
City: _____
State: _____ Zip Code: _____
Phone No: _____ Ext: _____
Fax No: _____

Employer: _____
Address: _____

## SUBJECTIVE COMPLAINTS

☐ Sharp pain in upper extremities
☐ Headaches ☐ right side ☐ left side ☐ increased ☐ decreased
☐ Facial paralysis ☐ dripping saliva ☐ increased ☐ decreased
☐ Ringing in ears ☐ hearing diminished ☐ increased ☐ decreased
☐ Eye pain ☐ right side ☐ left side ☐ watery eyes
☐ itchy eyes ☐ redness
☐ Thoracic outlet syndrome

☐ Carpal tunnel syndrome ☐ right hand ☐ left hand
☐ Hand pain ☐ right side ☐ left side ☐ increased ☐ decreased
☐ Numbness in fingers ☐ right side ☐ left side
☐ increased ☐ decreased
☐ Tingling in fingers ☐ right side ☐ left side ☐ increased ☐ decreased
☐ Tired arms ☐ weak arms

☐ Neck pain ☐ right side ☐ left side ☐ stiffness
☐ sharp pain ☐ decreased
☐ Restricted neck movement ☐ improved
☐ TMJ ☐ right side ☐ left side
☐ Shoulder tension ☐ right side ☐ left side ☐ increased ☐ decreased
☐ Pain between shoulders ☐ increased ☐ decreased
☐ Rotator cuff tendonitis ☐ right side ☐ left side

☐ Upper back pain ☐ increased ☐ decreased
☐ Midback pain ☐ increased ☐ decreased
☐ Tennis elbow ☐ right side ☐ left side
☐ Golfer elbow ☐ right side ☐ left side
☐ Sharp pain in range of motion ☐ decreased
☐ Difficulty to sleep ☐ sleep improved ☐ sleep well

☐ Progress with treatment
☐ Patient is better overall
☐ Patient wears wrist splints ☐ stop wearing ☐ wears again
☐ Pain shifted to lower extremities

- ☐ Sharp pain in lower extremities
- ☐ Lower back pain ☐ right side ☐ left side ☐ increased ☐ decreased
- ☐ Leg pain ☐ right side ☐ left side ☐ increased ☐ decreased
- ☐ Hip pain ☐ right side ☐ left side ☐ increased ☐ decreased
- ☐ Groin pain ☐ right side ☐ left side ☐ increased ☐ decreased
- ☐ Sciatica ☐ right side ☐ left side ☐ increased ☐ decreased

- ☐ Thigh and hamstring pull ☐ right side ☐ left side
  ☐ increased ☐ decreased
- ☐ Knee pain ☐ right side ☐ left side ☐ increased ☐ decreased
- ☐ Calf muscle pull ☐ right side ☐ left side ☐ increased ☐ decreased
- ☐ Diabetic foot pain ☐ increased ☐ decreased
- ☐ Ankle sprain ☐ right side ☐ left side ☐ swelling
- ☐ Tarsal tunnel syndrome ☐ right side ☐ left side

- ☐ Plantar-fasciitis and heel spurs ☐ right side ☐ left side
- ☐ Foot numbness ☐ right side ☐ left side
- ☐ Tingling (needle-prick feeling) in foot ☐ right side ☐ left side
- ☐ Tired feet ☐ coldness
- ☐ Difficulty in walking ☐ using stick ☐ walker ☐ cane
  ☐ crutches ☐ wheelchair
- ☐ Anxiety ☐ nausea ☐ dizziness ☐ irritability ☐ weakness
- ☐ Fatigue ☐ poor circulation ☐ poor mobility

- ☐ Blood pressure ☐ high ☐ low
- ☐ Stroke ☐ paralysis
- ☐ Subluxation (misaligned vertebrae) pinched nerve
- ☐ Significant stiffness with bending ☐ stooping
- ☐ Increased in handicap due to pain
- ☐ Increased in exacerbated pain level

- ☐ This patient needs evaluation by medical doctor.
- ☐ This patient needs x-ray examination or MRI.
- ☐ Patient stops using over the counter pain medication.
- ☐ Patient stops using prescribed pain medication by his/her physician.
- ☐ Patient is using herbal medicine. ☐ Stop using herbal medicine.

- ☐ Pain level has decreased with treatment.
- ☐ Significant improvement with home exercise program.
- ☐ Improved in sexual function capacity with ability to obtain/maintain erection.
- ☐ Patient is happy with treatment.
- ☐ Patient statement: _____
  _____

## OBJECTIVE FINDINGS

- ☐ Obvious pain
- ☐ Patient can bend, twist, or change posture without sharp, sudden low-back pain.
- ☐ Significant loss of range of motion

## DIAGNOSIS

- ☐ See doctor's first report.   ☐ See Dr. _____ report dated _____
- ☐ Cervical sprain/strain       ☐ Lumbar sprain/strain
- ☐ Right midfoot sprain         ☐ Laxity of ligament
- ☐ Cervical radiculopathy       ☐ L/S radiculopathy

## TREATMENT PLAN

- ☐ Acupressure Therapy  ☐ Acupuncture  ☐ Martial Arts Medical Massage
- ☐ Medical Massage  ☐ Massage Therapy  ☐ Magneto Therapy  ☐ Shiatsu
- ☐ Tuina   ☐ Physiotherapy   ☐ Chiropractic   ☐ Yoga   ☐ Tai Chi
- ☐ Manual Therapy    ☐ Other: _____
- ☐ Patient needs MRI/MRA regarding thoracic outlet syndrome.
- ☐ Demonstrate home exercises to patient.
- ☐ Demonstrate seated/work exercises to patient.
- ☐ Observe therapeutic exercises of patient.
- ☐ Patient needs to ergonomically correct work station (desk/chair).
- ☐ Goal: decrease pain, increase functional capacity
- ☐ Goal: increase in capacity to sleep
- ☐ This office is requesting authorization for treatment to the insurance carrier at a frequency of _____ times per week for _____ weeks.

## WORK STATUS

☐ This patient has been instructed to remain off work until _____
☐ Return to work on _____

## RESTRICTIONS

☐ standing  ☐ sitting  ☐ bending  ☐ kneeling
☐ lifting  ☐ typing  ☐ use of hands
☐ No over-the-shoulder work

I declare under penalty of perjury that this report is true and correct to the best of my knowledge and belief.

_____
DR. NAEEM SHARIEFF
*Acupressure Specialist*

Executed at Los Angeles, California
Date: October 20, 2011

# Taxila Sports Injury Clinic

386 Ventura Blvd., Encino, CA 91436                    Tel: (818) 000-1234

---

November 30, 2011

Attorney Claudia Martinez
33 Ventura Blvd., Suite 92
Encino, CA 91436

Regarding : Arshad Bahadur
Date of Injury: 09/13/2010

Dear Attorney Martinez,

## REVIEW OF RECORDS

Pursuant to your request for the review of records from Mumtaz Medical Center, I am forwarding to the following report.

I've received a sheaf of records approximately half an inch thick from Mumtaz Medical Center. These cover multiple dates during the years 2010 and 2011.

2-7-11, Dr. Ali, chief complaint: follow-up for headache.

10-5-10, Dr. Ali, chief complaint: body pain secondary to motor vehicle accident, prescription refill for Robaxin.

10-4-10, Saba, physical therapist, diagnosis: right shoulder impingement. Additional dates of service for this diagnosis were 09-06-06, 09-18-06, and 09-27-10.

9-6-10, Dr. Ali and Saba, physical therapist, referral for physical therapy for right shoulder impingement. Chief complaint is right shoulder pain of four to five months' duration, insidious onset, tingling in the right hand for greater than one year, motor vehicle accident 9-3-06 with whole body pain. History of patient admission to hospital in July 06 secondary to elevated blood pressure, medications atenolol and no pain medications. Additional noting of dizziness with change in position.

10-19-10, Baig German, MD, dictation number 244-3468.

12-22-10, Dr. Ali, hypertension controlled.

7-1-10, Discharge summary, referral for outpatient vestibular rehabilitation and further physical therapy needed.

7-12-10, Dr. Ali, chief complaint, back pain and patient feels unable to work. Focus of back pain is thoracolumbar and lumbosacral. Diagnosis is hypertension, spinal stenosis, and disk disease.

6-16-10, Chief complaint, body pain and weakness. Rx Tylenol.

5-24-10, Dr. Ali, chief complaint, blood pressure checked, patient had very high blood pressure on 5-19-06, BP 142/82.

5-19-10, Dr. Westchester MD, Dale Memorial Hospital, EKG, diagnosis sinus bradycardia with sinus arrhythmia, T wave abnormality, abnormal EKG.

1-26-10, Mumtaz Medical Center, hearing evaluation report.

Undated, clinical progress record, handwritten record, difficult to read, pertains to headaches limiting patient's ability to function.

1-26-10, Dr. Jack MD, evaluation of the ears secondary to hearing loss.

1-24-10, Carol Peace, referral for audiology evaluation.

3-22-11, Dr. Andrew Berger, two-view chest x-rays, no significant findings.

10-2-10, Dr. Richard Harris, one-view portable chest x-ray, no significant findings.

10-2-10, Dr. Simons, CT scan of the head without contrast, no significant intracranial findings.

10-2-10, Dr. David, myocardial perfusion stress scan, negative test, unchanged from 12-31-02.

8-10-10, right shoulder x-rays, Dr. Michael Brook, normal right shoulder.

7-17-10, Dr. Anne King, MRI brain with a contrast, minimal age-related atrophy, a few punctate nonspecific white matter foci.

6-30-10, Dr. Gary Rider, CT scan with a contrast, mild to moderate cortical atrophy without intracranial hemorrhage. The indication for this test was a severe left-sided headache with right side of numbness.

4-27-10, Michael Brook MD, X-rays of the bilateral hands, mild degenerative changes primarily in the first carpometacarpal joints.

1-27-11, Lab report.

10-3-10, Lab report.

7-14-10, Lab report.

10-2-10, Lab report.

7-7-10, Lab report, Gram's stain of CSF secondary to suspected diagnosis of meningitis.

7-1-10 Lab report, chemistry, and hematology.

4-29-10, Lab report, chemistry, and endocrinology.

6-13-11, Dr. Mona, progress note, chief complaint: left-sided chest pain.

4-20-10, Baron Fry, PA, progress note, CPAP causing irritation to upper lip.

3-22-11, Baron Fry, PA, progress note CPAP causing irritation around the lips.

1-24-11, Dr. Sam, progress note, dizziness.

There are no other records from Mumtaz Medical Center to review.

If you have any additional questions pertaining to this records review, please feel free to contact this office.

Respectfully,

_____
Dr. Remy Sharieff
*Acupressure Specialist*

# Alien Pain Care Clinic ™

336 Huge Tree Street, West Hills, CA 91307　　　　Tel: (818) 000-1234

---

|  |  |
|---|---|
| Patient Name: | Raj Gupta |
| SSN: | xxx-xx-1234 |
| Examination: | Right-Side Paralysis |
| Referring Physician: | Dr. Khan |
| Examination Date: | 10/04/2011 |
| Today's Date: | 12/05/2011 |

Manual therapy for pain control.

## CLINICAL HISTORY

Mr. Gupta, a seventy-year-old East Indian male, got an attack of paralysis on the right side of the body (hemiplegia). His right arm and right foot were affected. He was taken from many places for treatment, but this was of no use. One of his neighbors suggested this clinic for magneto therapy, and the family brought him over here.

## DIAGNOSIS IMPRESSION

Right-side paralysis.

## METHOD APPLIED

North pole under the palm of the right hand and south pole under the sole of the right foot.

## TREATMENT PLAN

Three thousand gauss of high-powered magnets used in this treatment, which has a capacity to lift 10 kg of iron weight.

Magnetic water was prescribed on daily basis.
Treatment was twice a day for fifteen minutes each.
Massage therapy twice a week for sixty minutes.

## RESULTS

As a result of this treatment for about two months, weakness of the limbs reduced gradually without the use of electromagnets. Recovery period depends upon person to person. Some take a shorter period of time and some take a longer period of time.

Thank you for referring this patient.

_____

NAEEM SHARIEFF, MDAM

# Alien Pain Care Clinic ™

336 Huge Tree Street, West Hills, CA 91307        Tel: (818) 000-1234

---

|  |  |
|---|---|
| Patient Name: | Sheila Petroman |
| SSN: | xxx-xx-1234 |
| Examination: | Thoracic Spine |
| Referring Physician: | Dr. Mehnaz Khan |
| Examination Date: | 06/12/2011 |
| Today's Date: | 07/24/2011 |

Manual therapy for pain control.

## CLINICAL HISTORY

Lower back pain. R/O disk herniation.

## TECHNIQUE

Martial arts medical massage was performed in chronic pain with the use of elbow, fingers, fist, and knuckles. The following methods were not used in this therapy: no electrical devices, no mechanical devices, no traction, no needles, no medications, no heat pad, no cold pad, no cupping, no heat lamp, no rollers and balls, no stones, no magnets, no laser, no ultrasound, no oil or lotion.

## FINDINGS

There is no abnormality noted or discovered.

## IMPRESSION

No disk bulging.

Thank you for referring this patient.

---

SHER SHAH SURI, LMT

# Alien Pain Care Clinic ™

336 Huge Tree Street, West Hills, CA 91307       Tel: (818) 000-1234

---

Patient Name:         Ganesh D' Souza
Date of Birth:        October 30, 2006
Examination:          Whole Body Paralysis
Examination Date:     10/31/2011
Today's Date:         12/05/2011

Manual therapy for paralysis.

## CLINICAL HISTORY

Ganesh D' Souza, a five-year-old Indian boy, was suffering from full body paralysis. He was brought by his mother to the clinic for treatment.

## DIAGNOSIS IMPRESSION

Whole body paralysis.

## METHOD APPLIED

Two different methods were applied for upper and lower extremities.

<u>Upper Extremity</u>
North pole under the palm of the right hand and south pole under the palm of the left hand.

<u>Lower Extremity</u>
North pole under the sole of the right foot and south pole under the sole of the left foot.

## TREATMENT PLAN

1. One thousand five hundred gauss of medium-powered magnets were used in this treatment, which is suggested for children between the ages of three to sixteen. It has a capacity to lift 5 kg of iron weight.
2. Magnetic water was prescribed three times a day, 1 oz., or 25 mL, at a time before breakfast and after a big meal.
3. Treatment was started twice a day for fifteen minutes then gradually increased to thirty minutes for faster recovery.
4. Physiotherapy on a regular basis.
5. Massage therapy on a daily basis.

## RESULTS

The patient has recovered within a month.

## DISCUSSION

Magneto therapy is an external treatment. It produces heat in the body and provides strength to the ten anatomical systems, such as circulatory system, nervous system, etc. A number of ailments could be cured by applying magnets. Therefore, it has been gaining popularity in many countries, including Russia and America.

Acupuncture points could be used as magnetic points for application of magnets <u>on</u> or <u>near</u> the selected points.

In this case, we used multiple points of hands and feet. If this is a matter of arthritis of hands and feet, same treatment would be recommended.

Magnetic water plays an important role. Scientifically, the properties of water change when it is polarized or magnetized and are beneficial to the health.

## DECLARATION

I declare that the information provided herein is true and correct to the best of my knowledge and belief.

_____

NAEEM SHARIEFF, MDAM

Enclosure(s): Images of treatment

## Images of Therapy

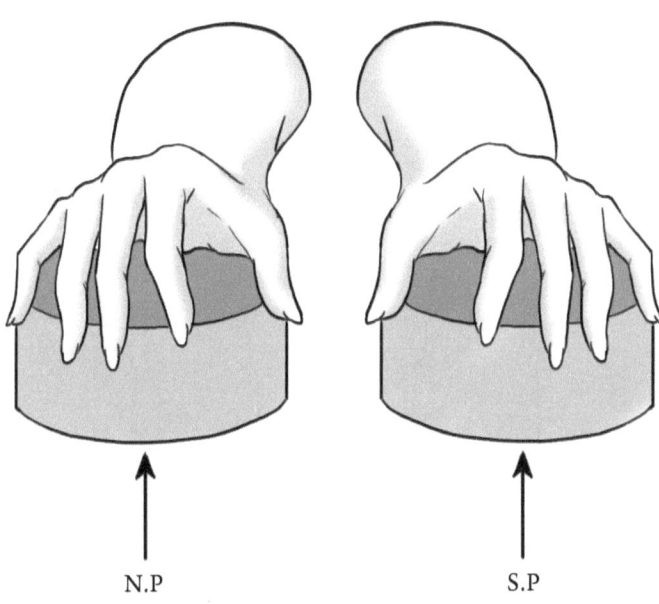

N.P                                S.P

**Figure 1**

# Images of Therapy

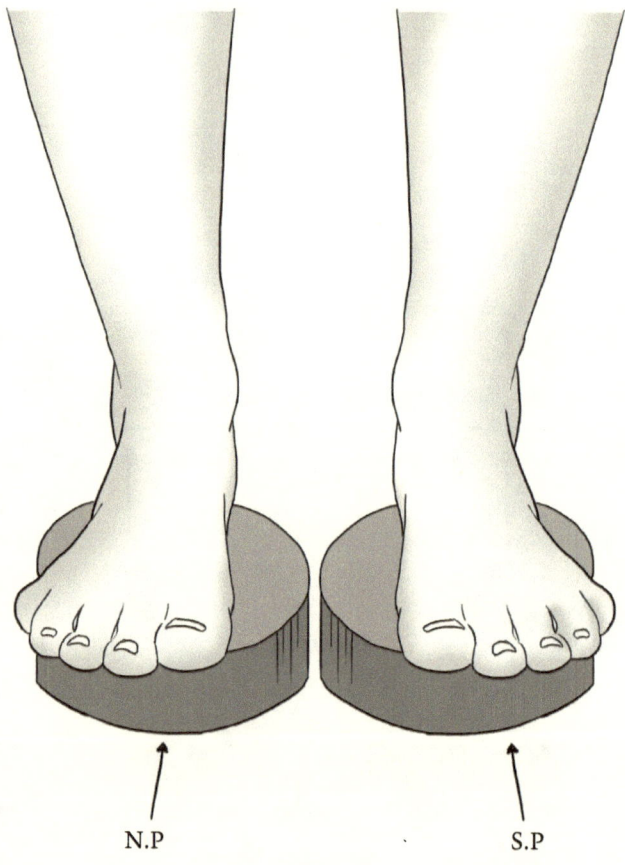

N.P           S.P

**Figure 2**

## Bonus Templates

| Sr. No | Topic | Page No. |
|---|---|---|
| 1. | Insurance Carrier Call-Tracking Record | 107 |
| 2. | Request for Release of Medical Records | 108 |
| 3. | Patient Appointment Calendar | 109 |
| 4. | Patient Visit Record | 110 |

## **Important**

Track communications with the insurance company. Keeping track of your phone calls can help you if you are ever denied payment, as some states and insurance companies will pay you if you can prove you were given an authorization of treatment.

# Insurance Carrier Call-Tracking Record

Patient Name: _____
SSN: _____ Account No: _____
Insurance Carrier: _____
Address: _____
Claim No: _____
Case No: _____ ☐ WCAB ☐ Superior Court
Claim Adjuster Name: _____
Phone No: _____ Ext: _____
Authorization Requested for: _____
Treatment Sessions: _____
Insurance Action: ☐ Accepted ☐ Denied ☐ Pending
What you need to do: _____
Follow-up schedule: _____
Date: _____
Day: _____
Time: _____
Caller Name: _____

# REQUEST FOR RELEASE OF MEDICAL RECORDS

Date: _____
Physician's Name: _____
Address: _____
Phone No: _____ Fax No: _____

I HEREBY REQUEST THAT MY MEDICAL RECORDS BE RELEASED TO THE FOLLOWING:
Medical Office: _____
Doctor's Name: _____
Address: _____
Phone No: _____ Fax No: _____

RECORDS TO BE DISCLOSED:
☐ Medical Report   ☐ Medical Legal Report   ☐ Medical Evaluation Report
Patient Name: _____
Address: _____
Date of Birth: _____ SSN: _____
Phone No: _____ E-mail: _____

Signature: _____ Date: _____
                    Patient/Legal Guardian

# PATIENT APPOINTMENT CALENDAR    JANUARY 2012

| Time | Sun 01 | Mon 02 | Tues 03 | We 04 | Thurs 05 | Fri 06 | Sat 07 |
|---|---|---|---|---|---|---|---|
| 09–10 | Ali | Ricky | Jim | Amina | Steve | Barbara | Areeba |
| 10–11 | Jon | Bob | | | Sergam | Moris | |
| 11–12 | Nuri | Khurshid | Chang | Nancy | Rim | Sam | |
| 12–1 | Tom | Abbas | | Suzuki | | | Zaheer |
| 1–2 | Hamid | Nasir | Lee | | Krulisky | | |
| 2–3 | | Cathy | Roger | Ayub | | Jose | |
| 3–4 | Irma | | | | Dona | | Kumar |
| 4–5 | | Lattie | Tony | Vicky | | Shakeel | |
| 5–6 | Sulaiman | | | Jimmy | Peter | | Poja |
| 6–7 | | Sehgal | Allan | | | Kim | Karla |
| 7–8 | Curtis | | Mo | Pervaz | Jacob | | |
| 8–9 | | Jakie | | | | Willis | Marshall |

Notes: _____

| Time | Sun 08 | Mon 09 | Tues 10 | We 11 | Thurs 12 | Fri 13 | Sat 14 |
|---|---|---|---|---|---|---|---|
| 09–10 | Nawaz | Buss | Gandhi | Altaf | Joe | Hussain | Shoib |
| 10–11 | Asif | Patty | | | Judy | | |
| 11–12 | | | Lisa | Karim | Ponce | Sham | Delip |
| 12–1 | Amir | | | | | | |
| 1–2 | | Khatak | Black | Yoko | | | Zamudio |
| 2–3 | | | | | | Ahmed | Reena |
| 3–4 | Norris | | | Abdul | Abraham | | Karima |
| 4–5 | | Tina | | | | Danis | |
| 5–6 | Perveen | | | | Honda | | Jerry |
| 6–7 | | | | Chiang | | Randi | Rani |
| 7–8 | | David | | | Ponam | Indra | |
| 8–9 | Khan | | | Bakir | | | Zuli |

Notes: _____

# Patient Visit Record

Name: _____ File No: _____

Date:_____ Day:____ Time In:_____ Time Out:_____ Session ☐ 30 min. ☐ 60 min.
Date:_____ Day:____ Time In:_____ Time Out:_____ Session ☐ 30 min. ☐ 60 min.
Date:_____ Day:____ Time In:_____ Time Out:_____ Session ☐ 30 min. ☐ 60 min.
Date:_____ Day:____ Time In:_____ Time Out:_____ Session ☐ 30 min. ☐ 60 min.
Date:_____ Day:____ Time In:_____ Time Out:_____ Session ☐ 30 min. ☐ 60 min.
Date:_____ Day:____ Time In:_____ Time Out:_____ Session ☐ 30 min. ☐ 60 min.
Date:_____ Day:____ Time In:_____ Time Out:_____ Session ☐ 30 min. ☐ 60 min.
Date:_____ Day:____ Time In:_____ Time Out:_____ Session ☐ 30 min. ☐ 60 min.
Date:_____ Day:____ Time In:_____ Time Out:_____ Session ☐ 30 min. ☐ 60 min.
Date:_____ Day:____ Time In:_____ Time Out:_____ Session ☐ 30 min. ☐ 60 min.
Date:_____ Day:____ Time In:_____ Time Out:_____ Session ☐ 30 min. ☐ 60 min.
Date:_____ Day:____ Time In:_____ Time Out:_____ Session ☐ 30 min. ☐ 60 min.
Date:_____ Day:____ Time In:_____ Time Out:_____ Session ☐ 30 min. ☐ 60 min.
Date:_____ Day:____ Time In:_____ Time Out:_____ Session ☐ 30 min. ☐ 60 min.
Date:_____ Day:____ Time In:_____ Time Out:_____ Session ☐ 30 min. ☐ 60 min.
Date:_____ Day:____ Time In:_____ Time Out:_____ Session ☐ 30 min. ☐ 60 min.
Date:_____ Day:____ Time In:_____ Time Out:_____ Session ☐ 30 min. ☐ 60 min.
Date:_____ Day:____ Time In:_____ Time Out:_____ Session ☐ 30 min. ☐ 60 min.
Date:_____ Day:____ Time In:_____ Time Out:_____ Session ☐ 30 min. ☐ 60 min.

## About the Author

The author has had a varied career in law, teaching, and research. He currently works as an alternative medical practitioner at Kung Fu Acupressure Therapy LLC in Los Angeles, California.

In 2011 he was awarded the gold award for his outstanding achievements in traditional martial arts and medicine by the World Culture Economic Trade Federation, Asian American Federation, and American Chinese Martial Arts Federation in the 13th World Cup Martial Arts Championship held at Los Angeles, California.

The author believes that this handbook, which is a compilation of case reports, would help the massage therapists and alternative medicine practitioners in writing medical reports for submission to medical-allied specialty or insurance carriers and good for educational and training purposes.

www.ingramcontent.com/pod-product-compliance
Lightning Source LLC
Chambersburg PA
CBHW030842180526
45163CB00004B/1426